TAPPING INTO *THE WIRE*

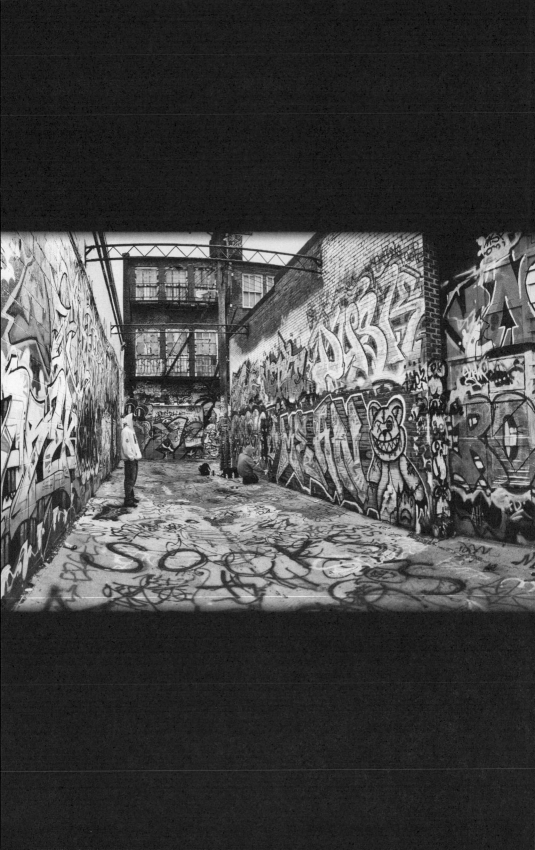

TAPPING INTO

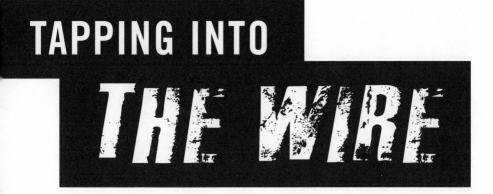

THE WIRE

THE REAL URBAN CRISIS

Peter L. Beilenson, M.D., M.P.H., and Patrick A. McGuire

Featuring a Conversation with David Simon

THE JOHNS HOPKINS UNIVERSITY PRESS

BALTIMORE

© 2012 The Johns Hopkins University Press
All rights reserved. Published 2012
Printed in the United States of America on acid-free paper
9 8 7 6 5 4 3 2 1

The Johns Hopkins University Press
2715 North Charles Street
Baltimore, Maryland 21218-4363
www.press.jhu.edu

Library of Congress Cataloging-in-Publication Data

Beilenson, Peter L.
    Tapping into The Wire : the real urban crisis / Peter L. Beilenson and Patrick A. McGuire ;
featuring a conversation with David Simon.
        p. ; cm.
    Includes bibliographical references and index.
    ISBN 978-1-4214-0750-0 (hdbk. : alk. paper)
    ISBN 1-4214-0750-7 (hdbk. : alk. paper)
    ISBN 978-1-4214-0761-6 (electronic)
    ISBN 1-4214-0761-2 (electronic)
    I. McGuire, Patrick A. (Patrick Anthony), 1946– II. Wire (Television program) III. Title.
    [DNLM: 1. Beilenson, Peter L. 2. Social Problems—Baltimore—Autobiography.
3. Urban Health—Baltimore—Autobiography. 4. Mass Media—Baltimore—Autobiography.
5. Public Policy—Baltimore—Autobiography. WA 380]
    362.1092'27526—dc23   2012008014

A catalog record for this book is available from the British Library.

Frontispiece: *Graffiti Alley, North Avenue at Howard Street,* Baltimore, 2011.
Photo: J. M. Fragomeni

*Special discounts are available for bulk purchases of this book. For more information,
please contact Special Sales at 410-516-6936 or specialsales@press.jhu.edu.*

The Johns Hopkins University Press uses environmentally friendly book materials,
including recycled text paper that is composed of at least 30 percent post-consumer waste,
whenever possible.

For my wife, Chris
and my children, Valerie, Alex, Jane, Jack, and Hank
for their constant support
and
my parents, Tony and Dolores
for their embodiment of principled public service

PB

For Kath

PM

CONTENTS

FOREWORD   A Conversation with David Simon,
Creator of *The Wire,* by Patrick A. McGuire   ix

CHAPTER 1   The New Public Health Crisis:
Wallace's World   3

CHAPTER 2   Heroin Central: *The Street Life of
Bubbles, Marlo, and Johnny*   19

CHAPTER 3   Losing the War on Drugs:
The Pit versus the Police   33

CHAPTER 4   Medicalize or Legalize: *Hamsterdam*   47

CHAPTER 5   Needle Exchange and the AIDS Dilemma:
Sticking It to "the Bug"   61

CHAPTER 6   Treatment on Demand as a Strategy:
Walon's Success Story   77

CHAPTER 7   School Performance and the MIA Parent:
The Tragedy of Dukie's Education   93

CHAPTER 8   Teenage Pregnancy and STDs:
Shardene's Escape   109

CHAPTER 9   Firepower: *Snoop's Beretta, Avon's Heckler,*
             and Omar's Mossberg   123

CHAPTER 10   Place Matters: *Why Didn't Bodie Just Leave?*   135

CHAPTER 11   Of Paint and Guns: *Did Omar Die*
             of Lead Poisoning?   149

CHAPTER 12   Obese Yet Malnourished: *The Weighty*
             Contradiction of Prop Joe   161

CHAPTER 13   Public Health and Politics: *The Promise*
             and Peril of Tommy Carcetti   169

EPILOGUE   Learning from *The Wire: Practicing Politics*
             to Practice Medicine   179

CAST OF CHARACTERS   189
NOTES   193
INDEX   207

A CONVERSATION WITH DAVID SIMON, CREATOR OF *THE WIRE*

by Patrick A. McGuire

AMONG THE THOUSANDS INSPIRED to enter journalism by the 1972 Watergate reporting of Bob Woodward and Carl Bernstein was a young, Bethesda, Maryland, teenager named David Simon. A writer for his high school paper and, later, editor of the *Diamondback* at the University of Maryland, Simon pursued his dream of becoming a reporter steadily and efficiently. He joined the staff of the Baltimore *Sun* only ten years later, in 1982. For most of the next thirteen years, he covered the paper's police beat.

The cop shop is not a glamorous reporting assignment. It is safe to say that most reporters who have covered the police department were not sad to leave it behind for something less chaotic and more predictable. The hours are awful, weekend shifts and night shifts are plentiful, and the information surrounding most crime stories is maddeningly difficult to pry loose from suspicious or personality challenged cops.

Simon, however, thrived at it, turning in solid copy marked by numerous inside sources and a gritty, readable style. He earned the trust of enough local cops that the department allowed him to spend a year practically living with the homicide squad while researching a book. When it was published, *Homicide: A Year on the Killing Streets* was grabbed up by

Baltimore native Barry Levinson, who turned it into an award-winning TV series with Simon writing many of the scripts.

During his newspaper days, it was clear to the reporters who worked with him—myself included—that Simon was a different breed of journalist. Besides being a tenacious reporter who knew how to get information, he was a writer of evocative prose. Sometimes forgotten is the notion that a journalist is one who strives to master two arts: reporting *and* writing. Often, those who approach such mastery are known by their passion—not merely for the job, for the career, or even for the paper. Rather, it's a passion for telling a story well. David seemed always ablaze with the righteousness of whatever story he was working on. He would defend his ideas long and hard against editors who thought they could impose their own vision of the story on him.

In my view, the Baltimore *Sun* was never a writer's paper. It was not the paper of H. L. Mencken—that was the *Evening Sun*, the afternoon paper that eventually died or was killed off, depending on how close you were to the body on the sidewalk. The morning paper, simply *The Sun*, proudly waved the banner of hard, serious news; it stood proud, sometimes to the point of overbearance, behind its laudable record in covering wars and international intrigue. It never quite figured out what it had in Simon or how to deal with his ever-broadening streak of independence. That he would one day leave seemed inevitable to many and became fact in 1995.

That year, Simon teamed up with former Baltimore homicide detective Ed Burns to write *The Corner*. It's a true-life look at an impoverished family living near the corner of Fayette Street and North Monroe—the heart of the west Baltimore drug world where dealers often sell their goods from street corners. Simon adapted the book into a six part mini-series for HBO. He wrote five of the six scripts and earned a credit as a producer. The series won three Emmy awards.

Simon then conceived the idea for a new HBO series called *The Wire* and was given the go-ahead to film a pilot. Again, he teamed up with writing partner Ed Burns. The series, which ran for five seasons, premiered on HBO in 2002. It introduced the world not only to Baltimore—its cops, politicians, drug addicts, union leaders, crime lords, and newspaper editors—but also to the state of crime, poverty, official indifference, and general urban decay found in most American cities. Its characters were fictional but drawn from the street reality Simon and Burns had observed and interacted with for years as newsman and detective.

Following that success Simon produced and wrote *Generation Kill*, a six-part HBO series based on a book of the same title by Evan Wright. It told the story of the First Reconnaissance Marine battalion during the 2003 Iraq invasion. His latest work for HBO, a series called *Treme*, focuses on a group of New Orleans musicians whose lives were dramatically affected by Hurricane Katrina.

In 2009, after Peter Beilenson asked me to join him in writing this book, I suggested that it include the voice of David Simon. In the fall of 2010, I interviewed David at his home in Baltimore's Locust Point. What follows are the highlights of that talk as they relate to the subject of this book: public health imperatives that are at the heart of every episode of the program David Simon called *The Wire*.

Patrick A. McGuire

Patrick McGuire: A relatively new model of public health is taking hold in many areas of the country. It goes beyond the traditional role of dealing with issues such as immunizations and safe-water initiatives. It views the spillover effects of drug-related chaos in our inner cities as a threat to the health and well-being of all citizens—not just those in certain neighborhoods. *The Wire* seems to mirror this view in depicting poverty, gun violence, and addiction as unsolved problems of public health and not just criminal justice. Was that an intentional focus?

David Simon: We made those points in *The Corner*. Since it was nonfiction, we made a much more fundamental argument in that show. *The Corner* was the reporting, whereas *The Wire* was like a big op-ed piece.

I remember having lunch with Peter Beilenson and Kurt Schmoke in the late nineties. Schmoke had read *The Corner* and asked to meet with Ed Burns and me. Schmoke basically said, "You guys get it. This is why I came out for decriminalization." I told him he was a prophet without honor in his own country. In many ways Schmoke was a pragmatic man in terms of filling potholes and getting stuff done and getting everyone moving the city forward. A little ethereal. He would have made a great senator. Being mayor is a much more prosaic thing. But as an idea guy he was smart as a whip.

Schmoke started to sour on the drug war with the killing of narcotics detective Marty Ward in '84. The guy who hit all over him for suggesting a discussion about decriminalization was Congressman Charlie Rangel. He wasn't addressing himself to what Schmoke was saying, which was absolutely accurate. He wasn't offering any other solutions and wasn't accepting the notion that the War on Drugs wasn't working. He savaged Schmoke.

THE CORNER WAS THE REPORTING, WHEREAS *THE WIRE* WAS LIKE A BIG OP-ED PIECE

At the time I thought, "Wow, Schmoke just wants to talk about it but we can't even talk about it." I don't know that I was as confirmed in my belief then that the drug war had to end. I was working on *Homicide*. I was surrounded by guys who were working drug-related murders. I didn't really start thinking about it until 1993–95 when I was researching *The Corner*. And then, all of a sudden, what Schmoke had said and done was prescient. In *The Corner*, we basically said it's an intractable war and unwinnable, it's destroying police work, destroying health initiatives. It's not succeeding.

PM: The theme of *The Wire* seems to be the inability of our public institutions to function without corruption, self-interest, or a political motivation behind every turn of a wheel. When you initially conceived the idea of *The Wire*, had you already decided which institutions to go after?

DS: First, I needed to see if HBO liked it. They only asked for the one season. It was entirely possible we would have only one season. I knew that we only had room enough in that one season to start an argument about undoing the drug war. Once they asked us, "Do you want to come back? Do you have more?" we said absolutely.

At that moment we could open it up and go into different things. So then there was a discussion with writers—myself and Ed Burns and later George Pelecanos, who was extremely influential. Richard Price kicked in after Season 3. We threw it open to the idea of what would we need to do to paint the city. The second season I was adamant about going to the port. Underlying all of that was reforming the underclass, which effectively is the drug war. That needed to be the second season.

The third season needed to introduce the political infrastructure because we needed that in place to speak to reform. We also needed in place somewhere in the series the futility of any attempt to reform the school system or address the school system. You could see the inertia there. And then the last piece had to be the media. Because you basically wanted to say, as a coda to the piece, by the way if you thought any of the problems that we've depicted are going to be addressed, the external watchdog has no teeth anymore.

So those were the five seasons, if we got five. We still had to beg. They gave us two and three pretty easily. We were almost canceled after three. Four was a hard fight. A lot of begging. After four there was talk about canceling the last season. It wasn't a hit. They had a limited production budget. They said, "We'll give you money to try something else, to shoot a pilot." They were looking for another *Sopranos*, and they said, "Why don't you take another shot at having a hit?" I kept saying, "I don't do hit." And then it turned out that *The Wire* became *The Wire*. Somewhere around the end of the fourth season the DVDs began to sell incredibly well. And they continue to sell to this day. Overseas it's huge. Nobody had seen that. I certainly hadn't. I didn't know people would want to watch it that way. Anyway they gave us a fifth season.

David Mills came in later and said, "Why don't you do something about the Latinos coming into Upper Fells Point?" *Immigration.* He was dead right. As soon as he said it I realized it was one that we'd missed. By the time he said it we were gearing up to do season four with the young kids—which also started the rise of Marlo's crew. It was a two year story arc, and we'd already planned the ending. Immigration is the one I wish we had done.

PM: What advantage did your background as a police reporter give you in writing *The Wire*?

DS: The *Sun* gave me an opportunity to observe at every level the systemic roots of an issue. I joke that my great success was never having been promoted at the *Sun*. I was always a police reporter. I covered the same things for thirteen years. Most of my shifts were shifts of rewrite and of police. In 1985 they were going to send me to Howard County. I said, don't let them send me out there. I refused, but that's like refusing the way out of the cops beat. Not the best career move. Once you cover counties well, you're maybe asked to be the third guy covering the legislature. Then maybe you work your way up to covering the state house. Maybe you get into the Washington bureau.

The problem with most police reporting is that people want to get off the beat. So, typically, you only cover the beat long enough to have written the usual eighteen-inch stories. Stories about cops showing the dope on the table after a police drug raid. And police reporters would cover it straight—as opposed to saying to themselves, "Wait a second. I've seen this for six or seven years, the drugs on the table. In fact, the corners are only getting worse. Drugs on the table don't matter."

So readers would get the same institutional dog and pony show and there would never be depth reporting on the drug war. Or what policing had become. Policing was being destroyed. The police department was learning mediocrity and learning stat work because what they were abandoning was police work.

By letting me into the homicide unit for the book *Homicide: A Year on the Killing Streets*, I met three hundred to four hundred cops. I had phone numbers and beeper numbers for half of them. The best of them were being wearied by the transformation in the police department. Not all of them agreed with me about the drug war, but all of them certainly agreed with me that the level of professionalism was dying. And they couldn't quite understand why. Some of them clearly understood that the easiest thing in the world is a drug arrest. And so you don't need to learn to do police work. Which is exactly what happened in the Baltimore police department. They raised generations of cops who didn't know how to make a case. Because you're not making a case. You're going out on the streets to get stats, whether or not those cases were ever prosecuted—that was not even of interest.

I stayed on the beat long enough that they couldn't wheel out the same old bullshit.

PM: *The Wire* starts out as a police story, but it quickly becomes much more than that, touching heavily on social issues. How did your social consciousness evolve?

DS: There's an ennobled version of me out there on the Internet that gives me too much credit. To me it's not social conscience. I just don't think of it in those terms. *The Wire* was getting all of the stuff you couldn't get into the paper and doing it with narrative forms and fictional storytelling. It's like reporters sitting around complaining about the things you can't get into the newspaper because those things are "editorial" in nature. The kind of stuff you tell each other over lunch. You tell each other the truth about what the mayor's really like or the truth over the flummery of what some institution is claiming as progress. Proving a lot of this stuff, particularly the personal stuff about people—especially the personal ambitions of people—is the hardest thing in journalism.

There was a police commissioner who was a genuinely good soul but who was not equipped to run a police department. And everybody knew he didn't have the acuity to run the police department. To be able to write that in a newspaper story would be epic. Or to write that another commissioner was going senile and would forget where he was and that people covered for him. These stories were throughout the department.

There was a story about these two high-ranking cops who hated each other. They were in competition for rank. One day one of them was the duty officer and he went out and saw that the word "police" was written backwards on the front of an emergency vehicle. And he called up the guy responsible and said, "I got you. You fucked this one up." That guy told him they write it backwards so that in your rearview mirror it reads frontwards. And the first guy says, "Oh, you got an answer for everything." That's the guy they made the police commissioner.

There's no way you can put that in the paper. The paper is fearful of being seen as opinionated. Or making a qualitative judgment like saying that the drug war doesn't work. That would be "provocative." The attitude was "you can't say that." I said, "Well, why not? I've been covering it for ten years." But you can say it in a TV show.

Everybody grafts onto me a motive because just telling a good story is never enough for people. So I'm either civic minded and socially responsible and passionate about those things (which I don't feel unpassionate about). But I never expected the world to get fixed. I came from a place where you tell a story and if it's shocking enough they pass a law and they make it worse. Telling a good story is the end in itself. And if something magical happened and they say we all watched *The Wire* and we're going to end the drug war because this is a disaster, then great. But it's never the expected result and not the intention. It was just a good story.

PM: Our current War on Drugs started out as a national policy. Do you think we'll invent a new national policy to replace it? Can the drug issue be resolved without a national policy?

DS: People are going to have to lead. I don't think there is political leadership. That sounds like pontification. Ed Burns had a great line. In order to lead you need to plant olive trees. You plant olive trees, and seven years later they give you the first crop of olives. There's no incentive if you're a politician on a four year election cycle to do that. Schmoke proved that. He proved there's no incentive. O'Malley learned the lesson well, and he has ascended and everyone who pretends to be tough on crime and tough on drugs has ascended.

I had lunch with Senator Jim Webb recently. His son was in Afghanistan, and when he came back he shoved *The Wire* at his father. Webb has since sponsored legislation trying to rationalize drugs. He's not for decriminalization. But he said we are the jailingest country in the world. We have put more people in prison and more per capita, more of a percentage of our people than China. More bodies. We're either the most evil people on the planet or something is really, really wrong.

What it is, is a war on the underclass and it will probably require a Republican president to say, "This is dumb. We're going to have jail cells for people we really need them for." When you target violent offenders and ignore the drug use, your crime rate goes down. You're taking people off the street who are violent. Most people who have drug problems are not violent. The average heroin user goes to work and cuts meat. At lunchtime he gets paid in cash because his boss knows he's a good meat cutter but has a problem. He gets a shot to maintain and gets paid the rest at the end of the day.

Heroin users are one of the most docile population groups. The violence is related by and large to the gangsterism that is a direct result of the illegality, not to the usage. Yes, there are people who go on a coke binge and end up shooting the mailman. But they're already violent. And I'm not suggesting there are good drugs. They are a disaster for people. But this notion that we are locking them up for drugs . . . First of all you can't hold

TELLING A GOOD STORY IS THE END IN ITSELF

them for drugs, because there's no room for them. If you lock up ten drug users, you'll get seven genuinely nonviolent people. Maybe two and a half people who can make a car radio disappear in a heartbeat and maybe half a soul who'll take a gun to somebody's head.

When somebody finds a way out, or someone takes pity on someone and gives them a job, that person is held up as "See you *can* get out, look at this guy who got out." But the validation of anybody as a human being allows you to be inhuman to everybody else. It's the moral equivalent to saying, "Some of my best friends are black." Or "There's a black family down the street and my kids play with their kids." We're past race—well, not everyone—but not past class. Class is huge. It's not that they're born black in the inner city; it's that they're being born poor. And white kids in Pigtown, they're as fundamentally extraneous and irrelevant as the black kids.

This is about class. In 1980 we started believing that if it makes money it's good. If it doesn't make money, why is government doing it? And that is a perfectly good way to maximize short-term profit. But it's not a good way to build a just society.

PM: Why did you cast Kurt Schmoke as the public health commissioner on *The Wire*?

DS: It was honoring Schmoke as a prophet. We were doing Hamsterdam and focusing on the idea of harm reduction. Schmoke's character was arguing that if we're gonna do this, let's put the health department into that area and do a needle exchange. Do outreach, so if people want to come off corners for treatment we can help them. It was the argument for harm reduction. I guess that was Beilenson's great ambition: to rationalize the reality, to make it coherent with what was possible and what was not.

PM: Among all the lines you wrote for *The Wire*, which is your favorite?

DS: My favorite line was something in Season 5 that, when I saw how good the director had set up a shot, I wrote it right on the set. The camera was panning these people who had been arrested. And they're all waiting on the bench to be processed. The camera is following Wendell Pierce, who plays Detective Bunk Moreland. And you see Squeak, this woman harridan. She was the one who was driving around to buy the cell phones with her boyfriend Bernard. And you see her on camera saying to Bernard, "You are the dumbest motherfucker." Originally that was the only scripted line. But on the day of shooting, I said once the camera is off Bernard, I want to hear him say, "I can't wait to go to jail." When we were editing it, I just laughed out loud. And then we brought Squeak back in and we had her say, "You did not just say what I thought you did."

In terms of a dramatic line that speaks to the whole theme: in Season 2 there's a scene where Frank Sobatka is talking to the lobbyist he bribed to get a measure passed in the state legislature. This is when Sobatka's learning that his ambitions are not going to get to the legislature. He says, "We used to make shit in this country. We use to build shit. Now we just put our hand in the next guy's pocket."

When we wrote that, the WorldCom scandal had just happened. I was writing a sort of generalist feeling about the unease with the economy. We wrote that scene two years before the collapse of the economy. Looking at what the mortgage bubble was and what Wall Street did to the world economy, that line makes us sound smarter than we are.

TAPPING INTO *THE WIRE*

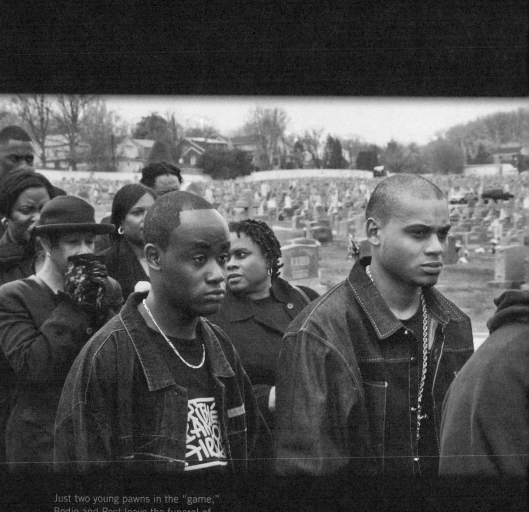

Just two young pawns in the "game,"
Bodie and Poot leave the funeral of
one of the many who died in the War
on Drugs in the acclaimed television
series *The Wire*. The series shows
the many casualties of this war, both
those who lose their lives and the
often neglected children that they
leave behind. THE WIRE/HBO ©

CHAPTER 1

THE NEW PUBLIC HEALTH CRISIS

WALLACE'S WORLD

MCKEAN AVENUE IS ONE OF BALTIMORE'S shorter streets, only four blocks long. It is sandwiched between two busy thoroughfares, a block east of North Monroe Street and just one block west of North Fulton Avenue. For decades in the early 1900s, Fulton was the westernmost border of a legally sanctioned zone of segregation—the only area in the city where blacks were allowed to live.

Though Baltimore's segregation laws were overturned long ago, an unofficial discrimination continued well into the twentieth century. By the 1930s, blacks represented one-fifth of the city's population, but they were confined to 2 percent of the city's area. After World War II, thousands of blacks migrated north from southern states and settled in the city to look for work. Black neighborhoods, already overcrowded, began a slow expansion in all directions as more and more families, mostly white, moved to the suburbs. Despite these changes, the heart of those old zones of segregation became the place where federal money built high-rise towers and low-rise, low-income housing projects. By the end of the last century, the only things that really thrived in those neighborhoods were poverty and drug addiction.

It may give you some sense of the saturation level of drug dealing in Baltimore to know that, in the first years of the new millennium, a drug gang led by a fourteen-year-old boy named Corey did not even control all four blocks of McKean Avenue. Yet the gang proudly laid claim to its small piece of turf with a name of almost innocent bravado: the Top of McKean Avenue Boys.

Those were the days when drug runners communicated with each other by pager, a system that soon evolved to using cell phones. Once the police proved capable of wiretapping even those, gangs moved to disposable cell phones, or "burners," which are much more difficult to trace. Corey, though, carried his pager proudly, and, caught up in running his gang, he skipped school 90 percent of the time. He lived in a dilapidated row house with his younger half-brother and his maternal grandmother. In the chill of November, the electricity had been turned off because they couldn't pay the bill. A space heater provided the only warmth, run with an extension cord that snaked out the front door of Corey's row house to an outlet in the equally seedy house next door.

Hopelessly ensnared in the often violent drug culture that pervaded Baltimore's inner city, Corey had a rap sheet that contained more than a dozen arrests. Corey's mother was long dead of AIDS, and his father was in prison in South Carolina on a drug charge. The grandmother he lived with was a heavy using, long-term heroin addict. As Corey's legal guardian, she was the beneficiary of a monthly social services check to cover the boys' needs. Most of that check went to support grandma's heroin habit.

My path first crossed with Corey's in 2002, my tenth year as Baltimore's commissioner of health. It was also the year that an HBO-TV series called *The Wire* began filming and showing its brutally realistic drama about Baltimore's drug culture. Not being an HBO subscriber, I knew the show only by the furor it caused in city hall, where its depiction of Baltimore's drug problem was viewed as a political negative.

I finally got around to watching the DVDs of *The Wire* a year after the show ceased production. I realized then that it was a perfect crystallization of all of the public health and social problems I had faced in real-life Baltimore during my thirteen years as health commissioner.

For instance, in the fall of 2002 the city's statistics for Corey's age group were alarming. The police had investigated thirty-two murders of juveniles, earning Baltimore the unenviable reputation as the city with the highest juvenile homicide rate in the country. Looking for ways to intervene, the Baltimore City Health Department reviewed every one of those homicide reports. What we found, while disturbing, was almost predictable. Of those thirty-two murders, all were committed with a gun. Among the victims, twenty-eight were boys and four were girls. All of the girls had been innocent bystanders, hit by errant bullets. All of the boys had multiple arrests for drug distribution and handgun violations. All of them had been shot at close range with large-bore weapons that imprinted the body with burn marks from the muzzle flash. Clearly, these murders were hits ordered by drug gang leaders.

In response, we started a program whose goal, I thought, was modest. As an urgent matter of public health, we set out to find the next thirty-two juvenile homicide victims in Baltimore—before they became victims. I would soon learn just how monumentally ambitious that idea was. Later, when I began watching *The Wire,* I realized that its producers, directors, and writers already knew that. And although those people had never met Corey, many of the characters portrayed on *The Wire* were very young teens, almost duplicate fictional versions of kids exactly like him.

UTTER THE WORDS "PUBLIC HEALTH" to almost anyone and watch their eyes glaze over. That's not the reaction you get when you talk about *The Wire,* which holds a viewer's attention as if at gunpoint. But this was not just a crime drama. In addition to portraying violence and drug dealing, it also concentrated on drug addiction and poverty with the kind of depth and realism that leaves stippling marks on the soul.

The Wire lays out social and environmental problems like an oil spill. What you see on the surface is the sheen from the underlying problems gushing upward and contaminating every aspect of civic life. In episode after brilliantly staged episode one sees instances of disintegrating fami-

> THE WIRE LAYS OUT SOCIAL AND ENVIRONMENTAL PROBLEMS LIKE AN OIL SPILL

lies, unchecked teen pregnancy, single-parent child rearing, homeless heroin addicts spreading AIDS through dirty needles, concentrated poverty, endless violence, the failure of schools, and the inability of the police to stop the drug trafficking.

If nothing else, *The Wire* is a microcosm of all the consequences of our country's failed War on Drugs: deep poverty and hopelessness and very little access to good jobs or a good education. When people don't have those things, they turn to drugs—either as users or dealers—and chaos follows. By the time I had seen the last episode, I knew *The Wire* was a perfect tool for changing perceptions and misconceptions about the deadly connections between drugs, crime, and poverty—as well as the role of public health in addressing them.

I knew very little about public health when I got out of medical school in the early 1990s. If I'd been asked to define it, I probably would have said it had to do with controlling diseases, providing immunizations, and safeguarding the food and water supply. Some public health officials today refuse to let go of that restrictive view. Certainly in the pecking order within the medical world, all rights to glamour and prestige (not to mention the lion's share of funding) go to those who provide specialized care to individuals—not to those who deal with the collective health of diverse populations.

Although it's not surprising that someone would have a limited view of public health, I do think that in today's world it's a mistake. My own definition—and that of many others tuned to the inevitable changes, both good and bad, that were wrought by twenty-first-century progress—incorporates social and environmental elements with traditional clinical health.

The guiding principles of public health are to promote health and to prevent unnecessary illness, injury, and death. If you look at it in terms of years of potential life lost, this construct begins to make sense. For instance, the average life expectancy in the United States in 2010 is just shy of seventy-eight years. But if you live in the inner city and die of AIDS at thirty-eight, that's forty years of potential life lost to you, your family, and society. That's not just theory. There are some parts of Baltimore's poverty-ridden inner city that statistically show a twenty-year lower life expectancy than in an upscale neighborhood such as Roland Park, just a couple of zip codes away. This new rationale of public health argues that attempting to modify social and environmental conditions to prevent early morbidity (the onset of significant illness or injury) and mortality (death) is as important to keeping people healthier and alive over the long run as promoting flu shots or treating wastewater to prevent typhoid.

AMERICA RISES AND FALLS with the health of its big cities. Although this country began as a predominantly agrarian society, it was only with the development of its large urban centers and their respective economic engines that the United States emerged as a major global economic and political power.

Even with today's suburbanization of America, the success of our large metropolitan areas hinges largely on the strength of the major cities they are centered on. Thus, metropolitan areas like those in northwest Washington state and eastern Massachusetts are doing well because of the generally sound economic and social health of Seattle and Boston, respectively. Other metropolitan areas, like those in south-central Michigan and northern New Jersey, have significant problems because of the economic and social challenges facing Detroit and Newark.

What many people do not realize is how much the economic and social strength of our major cities depends on the health of their citizens. But health can be broadly defined. Of course it includes the burden of chronic diseases and conditions like diabetes, hypertension, and obesity that can limit the ability of individuals to be fully employed, pay taxes, and function effectively in society. Those conditions also trigger the need for more local social and clinical services for the individuals afflicted.

But while violence, drug addiction, homelessness, and like conditions are not always viewed broadly as public health issues, their existence directly affects everything from the way a city is perceived nationally (cities with high crime rates are constantly held up as examples of failing urban areas), to the quality of its public schools (high rates of substance-abusing parents or school violence lead to middle-class flight from the school system), to its economic vitality (businesses and families are less likely to relocate to a city with substantial public health problems).

How a city addresses these major public health issues can make a big difference in its chances to successfully compete in challenging times as well as to improve the daily lives of its citizens. Since the early 1900s it has been the role of local public health agencies to take on this challenge. In the first half of the twentieth century, significant strides were made in public health—including widespread immunization and vastly improved sanitation practices—that have led to a dramatic increase in the average American's life expectancy.

In 1900, a baby born in the United States could expect to live to the age of forty-seven; a baby born in 1950 could expect to live to sixty-eight. And, as noted earlier, by 2010, life expectancy for an American baby had increased to seventy-eight years. Although such a phenomenal jump is unlikely to be repeated over a similar period of time, there is much we can do to improve the health of our citizens by using the first half of the twenty-first century to address a host of new public health challenges.

That is why drug abuse and the despair and violence it spawns are as much a health issue as the flu. Drug addiction is a chronic disease. It's not unlike high blood pressure or diabetes: you have it for a lifetime, you have relapses, your behavior is impacted, and ongoing treatment is needed. But there's a lot more stigma attached to being a substance abuser than to being a diabetic. Oddly, if you look at it in terms of an individual's compliance with treatment measures—drug abusers versus diabetics or those with high blood pressure—the substance abusers do better.

It's hard to argue against the main theme of *The Wire* that drug abuse and the violence it engenders foster serious social consequences. If a city doesn't deal with them effectively, it won't be long before related problems join them—absenteeism from work, kids not being ready to learn, and kids dropping out of school and causing violence.

Those who hold this broader view believe that practitioners and policy makers should cast a wide net to encompass the different aspects of public health. For example, racial relations become relevant and determine people's outcomes in life—not just vocational outcomes but their health. Another example of the expanded view of public health is taking into account the disparity in access to health care between the poorest and everyone else. That is why public health must be viewed as writ large rather than follow the circumscribed, old-fashioned model of standard communicable disease control.

ON THE SURFACE, CHARACTERS IN *The Wire* like Johnny and Bubs, Stringer and Avon, Bodie and Poot are fictions drawn from the imaginations of the program's creators. But the firsthand street experience of writers David Simon, a former Baltimore *Sun* police reporter, and Ed Burns, an ex–city school teacher and homicide detective, make it clear that the names of their characters are the only real fiction in the story.

When I watched the first season, I was particularly taken by the story of Wallace, one of the young teenage boys pushing heroin in the courtyard of the city's old low-income housing projects. He is portrayed as an innocent, a boy who grew into his teen years without parents, emerging into the only life he had ever known—the world of drugs. But his heart isn't in it, and he certainly isn't a good fit in this world. And that lands him in trouble.

There's a poignant scene in Episode 6, Season 1, in which Wallace wakes up one morning in a derelict row house surrounded by a passel of sleeping kids. They are much younger than he but, like him, they are kids without mothers or fathers. The scene opens with the camera following a very long electric cable that snakes across the backyards of other row houses and into Wallace's bedroom. This, we realize, is the only source of power in the house. As Wallace gets the younger kids ready for school, giving each a bag of chips and a juice box, police outside are examining the body of a man tortured to death by drug lords.

In a subsequent episode, after Wallace hides out on Maryland's rural Eastern Shore, he returns to his old city haunts. He is asked by a friend why he came back. I had to laugh at hearing this question, as you might as well ask Wallace why he couldn't have simply said no to drugs, gotten a job, worked hard, and gone to Harvard to become a brain surgeon. Wallace says something to the effect that this is his home; he is a corner boy, not a country boy, and that's who he will always be.

We know he speaks the truth, for at that young age, bereft of education, guidance, and opportunity, his future has been sealed irrevocably. At the end of the episode Wallace is murdered by two of his fellow crew members, both close friends who rationalize the killing by noting that Wallace had simply paid the price for screwing up.

During those episodes, I was struck by the eerie similarities between Wallace and the boy I've called Corey. Confidentiality laws prohibit me from using his real name and so, like Simon and Burns, I have made one up. Bear in mind, however, that Corey is a real boy who lived in a surreal world that few who live outside of it can imagine. And that's what jolted me. Watching *The Wire*, I realized Corey's story could easily have fit in as one of the many subplots of the series.

THE PLAN WE LAUNCHED IN 2002 was called Operation Safe Kids and was modeled after a similar program in Boston. The idea wasn't just to get kids treatment or counseling or a helping hand. What the thirty-two boys—whose names we did not yet know—needed went beyond normal interventions. Unless some big changes were made in their lives, each was a statistic waiting to be counted.

The plan called for an extraordinary level of cooperation across many city and state agencies. It required meaningful input from police, social services, the school system, the criminal justice system, and others. I think what ultimately made it successful was not simply getting such agencies to work together but getting high level leaders of each agency to sit together at a table once a week and, with no nonsense, work out a unique plan for each boy.

That we were able to convince those leaders to attend meetings every week had much to do with the ignominy of Baltimore's reputation regarding juvenile murder. But it also had a lot to do with helping each leader to see the value in this unusual plan. We could lower our homicide rate, yes, but literally we could save and rebuild the lives of severely troubled kids who were considered beyond help.

We started working with the Maryland Department of Juvenile Services (DJS) to establish criteria for exactly which teenage boys we were targeting. Then DJS, with the public defender's office and the Baltimore Police Department, identified juveniles who matched our criteria. Basically, we were seeking kids with multiple arrests for drug distribution and a history of handgun violence.

Corey was literally the first kid in the program. His case was presented to our group of agency leaders by a DJS probation officer and then turned over to one of our case managers.

We made it a point of recruiting our case managers from the very inner city communities we were targeting. We had learned, sometimes the hard way, that assuming people would trust counselors from outside their world was a formula for failure. At the same time, it was a disheartening fact of inner city life that many adults from those neighborhoods died prematurely in their fifties, often of cancer or diabetes. I remember particularly one of our case managers, a mother whose own child had been shot and killed on inner city streets. She was extremely effective as a case manager, but when she died suddenly at forty-nine, she looked sixty-five. Without doubt, there's a connection between shortened life expectancy, poverty, and difficult life circumstances.

The first thing our leadership group did was review Corey's immediate needs. We got the electricity in his house turned on. We got him food through various emergency programs. Still, his set-up was far from ideal. He wasn't going to school, and his grandmother needed treatment for her drug problem.

Corey's case manager offered the grandmother entry into a residential drug treatment program, but she refused. It turned out she was afraid of losing the money sent to her each month by social services for the guardianship of Corey. In the meantime we got Corey moved to a new home. He was taken in by his paternal, working-class grandparents. They were solid citizens and a courageous, remarkable couple. They lived in a well-kept row house in Fort Washington on the east side of Baltimore. They had never met Corey's maternal grandmother or his mother. But since Corey's father was their son who had fallen off the deep end, they were willing to take in not only Corey but the grandmother—if she got clean.

After two weeks of wrangling with Corey's grandmother, she agreed to enter a treatment program for heroin addiction. We worked it out with social services that she could keep getting the guardianship money for the time being. The result was that Corey got away from the people, places, and things on the west side of town that got him into trouble. In Baltimore, Charles Street separates the east and west sides of the city and is viewed with trepidation by drug gangs as the line of demarcation. The tradition—an outgrowth of the parochial nature of the city—held that corner boys from one side of the city never set foot on the other side. Thus, moving Corey across Charles Street to the east side was almost like sending him to a new country for a fresh start.

Things went well for a time. Corey was willing to take part in the program (his younger half-brother stayed on the west side with the boy's birth father). The city school system got Corey placed in a Fort Washington middle school. He was out of the drug trade. His grandmother eventually got clean and moved in with him and his other grandparents.

The city's police commissioner, Ed Norris (who later played a detective by the same name on *The Wire*), had given me a police pager so I could be notified of major crimes as they occurred. I didn't see any real use for it and mostly thought of it as a curious perk of the job. But one night three months later, in February 2003, I got a jolting page. A fourteen-year-old black male juvenile had been found shot to death on the west side. At first I breathed a sigh of relief because we didn't have many fourteen-year-olds in the program on that side of town. It didn't sound like any of our boys. Then I got a call from the woman who supervised our case managers. The dead boy was Corey.

We found out later that Corey had gone back to the west side to attend the birthday party for his half-brother. A thirteen-year-old boy who'd had a beef with Corey months back during his Top of McKean Avenue days saw him on the street and promptly shot him in the back.

Corey's death was tragic and discouraging. My immediate thought, beyond grief at the loss of another young life, was: here was a very expensive program with lots of high-level officials, from the police homicide division to the chief juvenile public defender, the chief of the juvenile division of the states attorney's office, the director for Region I of the Department of Juvenile Services, and more. Together we provided all of the services that a typical kid in trouble would not normally get to help solve his family problems. And yet with all of that, this tragedy still happened.

Several of us from the health department attended Corey's wake, held in a funeral home in a west side row house. As a city official, I'd attended quite a number of wakes and funerals, often witnessing spontaneous and understandable emotion. But not at this one.

When we arrived we found Corey's grandmother sitting on the front steps drinking out of a paper bag. With Corey dead, she had lost her principal source of income. Inside, the majority of the people in the crowded viewing room were teenage girls carrying babies. Most wore tee shirts that said "R.I.P. Corey" and listed his date of birth and death. It occurred to me that someone out there was making those tee shirts because there was a market for them and that this was not the first time such shirts had been ordered and worn. Nor would it be the last.

The dozens of teens making up the mourners chattered on cheerfully like it was a high school lunch hour—as if this wake was a common occurrence. No one seemed to be paying any attention to Corey, who lay in an open casket looking like a sweet, sleeping fourteen-year-old kid. A couple of boys trying to look tough stood in a corner dressed in trench coats and saying nothing. I wouldn't have been surprised at all to find out they were armed.

I remember projecting my own feelings of distress onto what I felt was a surreal experience. When I was eight years old, my fourteen-year-old neighbor died of leukemia, and it was a huge blow to me. It actually changed my life and made me want to go into medicine. I wondered how I would react had I been fourteen and Corey was my friend who'd been shot and killed. I knew I'd be devastated. Yet here, none of the mourners seemed devastated or even upset. This is exactly the dead-end atmosphere so honestly, and heartbreakingly, portrayed in *The Wire*.

While we were there, a pastor spoke, and then the funeral director. Finally a man who identified himself as Corey's father, freshly released from prison in South Carolina on a drug conviction, stood up. His first words were painful to hear. "I never met my son," he said, "but if I had, this is what I'd say to him . . ."

Sadly, this was a reality all too common. My thoughts went immediately to a study we had conducted sometime earlier. A striking number of the men in neighborhoods like Corey's who had fathered a child were at least ten to fifteen years older than the fourteen- to fifteen-year-old mothers-to-be. Plenty of them were twenty to thirty, even forty years older, men who obviously had taken advantage of these girls before disappearing from their lives. Another study showed that a stunning percentage of teenage mothers not only didn't know the fathers before becoming pregnant by them but never saw them after the birth, as was the case with Corey's parents.

Corey's father ended his brief remarks by calling for those present to spread the word: avenging Corey's death with more violence would solve nothing. "Please don't retaliate," he said. But only a couple of days later, the thirteen-year-old boy arrested for Corey's murder and then surprisingly released on bail was shot dead. His killers were Corey's cousin and a second boy. Not long after that, both of Corey's avengers were shot and the boy with the cousin that day was killed.

At that point, four months into Operation Safe Kids, we had identified and intervened—mostly successfully—in the lives of many boys like Corey. We would eventually top one hundred success stories before I left the city health department in 2005. Corey's would be the only instance of a tragic return to violence, and the memory of it still hurts.

I THINK AN INEVITABLE QUESTION one asks after viewing *The Wire* is, what would I have done? Had I grown up in that environment without parents, without knowing I'd have food every day, without the chance of a decent education, without knowing basic truths about the world around me (a *Wire* episode has corner boys marveling at the invention of Chicken McNuggets), without a guiding hand to point me in the right direction and advise me on right and wrong, with violence and fear being common occurrences, would I not seek out whatever support system was available that could provide for me? And if that support system was involved in the selling of drugs or killing those who stood in my way, and if I expected to be dead by twenty-five anyway (as so many corner boys casually predict of themselves), what realistic chance would I have of escaping that life?

There are many lessons to be learned from *The Wire*, and ever since viewing it I have sought to work those points home in the courses I teach at the Johns Hopkins University. It's not that *The Wire* presents solutions. The crime, poverty, and social chaos it depicts in Baltimore haven't gone away. In fact, many in Baltimore regard *The Wire* the way the city's mayor angrily responded during a cabinet meeting I attended in 2003. Martin O'Malley believed *The Wire* was a terrible program because, he said, as he was trying to make changes and improvements in the city, all that people anywhere knew about Baltimore was its drug problem.

Another take, however, is that because of its honesty and popularity *The Wire* has focused a bright light on serious problems—not just in Baltimore but any city with rampant poverty and drug-related crime. As long as that light is on (and fortunately *The Wire* continues to sell well in DVD long after its last episode was shown on HBO), an opportunity exists to use it to help change preconceived notions about poverty and drugs.

People *do* get it that crime is related to drugs and that we should provide treatment to nonviolent addicts. At the same time a prevailing attitude seems to be this: "Not in my backyard; get these people away from us; and do something about the crime." But no plan can expect much success without, at the very least, a begrudging awareness that stuffing prisons full of low-level drug users or dealers, almost all of them nonviolent offenders, has not worked.

A more realistic solution would be in everybody's best interest, but very few people have really thought about the benefits of a more practical approach. If you live in Baltimore's surrounding suburbs, then in order for the state to have the best economic engine it can have, you need to care that Baltimore City kids are achieving. At rock bottom it makes a real financial difference to you, so it's in your self-interest to want good city schools.

THE CITY BEHIND THE WIRE IS WHATEVER CITY YOU'RE IN OR NEAR RIGHT NOW AS YOU READ THIS

A large percentage of suburban dwellers in the Baltimore area—both black and white—came originally from the city. Among them I believe there remains a significant number who regard people like Corey, his grandmother, his murderer, and others like them with the complaint, "We pulled ourselves up by our bootstraps, why can't they?" Yet many of these same people diminish the importance of the strong family support systems that provided them their bootstraps to begin with. Antagonism toward those who need help spends a lot of energy but doesn't address the real problems, tending instead to demonize people and polarize the discussion.

I HOPE THAT IN THIS BOOK *The Wire* can be a road map for exploring the real-life connections between inner city poverty and drug-related violence. With a firm grip on the hard truths one can then take part in the serious dialogue that will lead to solutions.

Solutions, by the way, are not as simple as identifying what needs to be done. In my lectures I speak of the four-legged stool formula for a successful city. Such a city must have decent, affordable housing; available jobs with benefits that pay a livable wage; a more than adequate education system; and accessible health care and healthy food. The daunting task is negotiating the particular mechanics in politics and government for achieving each of those conditions. Even so, nothing will ever happen until misconceptions are replaced by understanding.

In a 2008 *TV Guide* interview, Michael Kenneth Williams, the actor who played the shotgun toting Omar Little, said, "I hope some kid in the 'hood will see *The Wire* and take a different turn. It isn't a white or black story. It isn't a Baltimore story. It's an American story. It's a social problem that's been going on in our country—though the country may not realize it."

So even though this roadmap bears the name of Baltimore and will focus on these problems in terms of our successes and failures in Baltimore, I tend to view the larger picture in terms of Everycity. In other words, in terms of public health, the city behind *The Wire* is whatever city you're in or near right now as you read this.

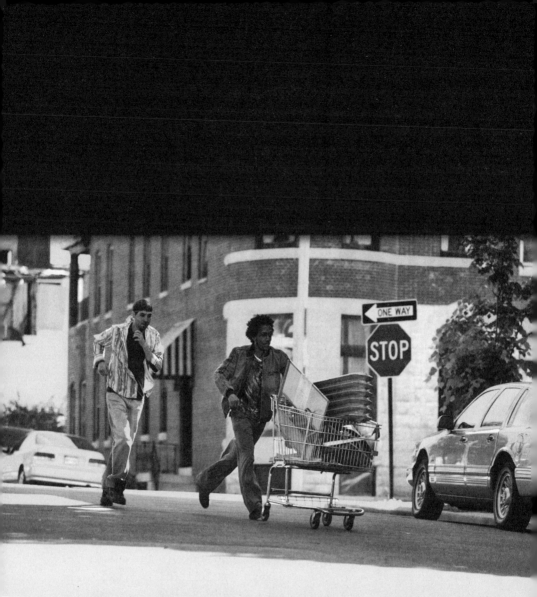

Bubs and Johnny collect busted
radiators and other trash that they
hope will provide enough cash
for their daily heroin fix. Billions
of dollars a year are spent buying
illegal drugs, with a significant
portion of the money coming
from selling stolen goods such
as these. THE WIRE/HBO ©

CHAPTER 2

HEROIN CENTRAL

THE STREET LIFE OF BUBBLES, MARLO, AND JOHNNY

I HAVE HEARD THE ARGUMENT dozens of times, and each time I cringe at its faulty simplicity: "Using drugs such as heroin and cocaine is illegal. So is selling these drugs on the street corners of our cities. Since these activities are illegal, there is no question about how we should respond to people who take part in such behavior—prosecute them and lock them up."

In many ways, the point of this book is to provide a rational response to that oft-repeated assertion. In my years working with people across the political spectrum in medicine, politics, public health, and academia, I have found that this view reflects a commonly held public perception and attitude about the drug problem facing America's cities. Unfortunately it misses the mark.

Much of this sentiment comes from both a frustration that things don't seem to be getting better in many cities and a lack of understanding of the life circumstances for so many of our fellow citizens living in dire straits. Sometimes, one person's belief about another person, an issue, or an event is based on a blunt but overly simplified judgment that doesn't really consider the whole story. Dispelling these simplistic concepts was one of the values I saw in *The Wire*.

The show takes as its starting point the idea that what we think we understand about people caught up in the world of drugs—who are the good guys and who are the bad guys—will become less and less clear the deeper we, as viewers, are exposed to them and their circumstances. *The Wire* is basically an in-depth look at the lives and motivations of various fictional characters who are working members of one of Baltimore's social institutions—such as the police department or the school system—whose purpose is to help the public. At the same time the series zeroes in on those members of the public who are to be served by these agencies, whether in the form of police protection, a well-rounded education, the competent running of a city government, or even the delivery of truthful news to assist people in making decisions about their well-being.

Finally, the show looks at those people who try to take advantage of a particular system, thereby corrupting themselves, others, and the entire rationale for that institution to exist. Over its five seasons, *The Wire* examines policing and the War on Drugs, the lack of jobs for the working class, politics, the social welfare and school systems, and journalism. Each themed episode is populated by the good, the bad, and the seriously bad. The most fascinating aspect of the entire series, however, is not just how difficult it is to separate the good guys from the bad, but how even though these people are made up, they resemble our own lives and the lives of those we all deal with or hear about on a daily basis.

While bad guys like Omar Little, a drug-connected assassin, and good guys like homicide detective Jimmy McNulty are invented characters, their words and actions are grounded in a familiar reality that is hard for anyone who has stood on a corner in west Baltimore to deny. Sometimes in *The Wire*, McNulty seems to be a little bit bad and sometimes Omar seems to be a little bit good. Sometimes it's hard to tell the difference between them and sometimes that doesn't seem to be the point anyway.

Squeezed in among scenes of violence in the third season of *The Wire*, a low-key moment of pathos and farce pops up that goes to this point and merits a closer look. It certainly illustrates for me how the problem of illegal drugs is not so easily consigned to one of crime and punishment.

In the scene, from Episode 26, Season 3, we zoom in on a pair of pitiful heroin addicts. Bubbles, who is black, and Johnny, who is white, are mindlessly pushing a stolen supermarket shopping cart in broad daylight down the middle of a west Baltimore street. In the cart, along with other stolen items they hope to sell for drug money, sits a stubby, accordion-like cast-iron radiator, plundered from a nearby vacant house.

When Bubbles and Johnny come to the top of a hill, the shopping cart and its sixty-pound weight eludes their grasp. It rolls unattended down the street and into a parked SUV. Turns out the vehicle is owned by one of the armed stooges loyal to Marlo Stanfield, the cold-blooded challenger to Avon Barksdale's heroin gang. The stooge—as mindless as the two addicts who come trotting down the road out of breath after their cart—scowls at the minor scrape on his truck. He is just turning his gun and murderous attention on Bubbles as Marlo emerges from a building. Viewing the pending killing of Bubbles, Marlo says in a bored voice, "Do it or don't. I've got someplace I gotta be." The next scene shows that Bubbles and Johnny survived their close call but are now pushing their cart while wearing only their underwear.

The scene contains many of the familiar beats of *The Wire*: hapless addicts, vicious drug dealers, a jolt of tension, a twinge of pity, and a leavening of humor.

If one simply applies the standard criminal scale to the four characters in this scene, they are prime examples of those who many feel should be locked away. That scene, however, gave me a deeper understanding. Beyond a simple picture of criminals bumbling into criminals, it showed a marked difference between a criminal with a gun and one without. That gun and the threat of violence immediately separate Marlo and his hired muscle from Bubbles and Johnny. They are of two different worlds. What we see here is a standoff between predator and prey, between the vicious and the broken. Certainly Marlo's contempt for Bubbles and Johnny doesn't make financial sense, since, without people like them, Marlo would be out of business. But just as a savage beast would as soon eat you as look at you, to a feral sociopath like Marlo business always takes a backseat to a show of power.

The scene conveys also a sickening sense of how one man's desperate need for the $50 or so it takes to supply his daily fix can degrade his existence into that of a groveling thief, willing to stoop low to fend off demons both within and without. Absent a close-up look at this sad reality, it is difficult to imagine one's own life so deteriorating into darkness that sense could be made of wrenching a sixty-pound cast-iron radiator from its moorings and placing it into a shopping cart on the chance it might bring $50. Yet mixed in with a viewer's revulsion at the pitiful person Bubbles has become, there brews a distinct understanding that he has not fallen nearly as far as Marlo.

In fact, given a chance at rehabilitation, nonviolent addicts like Bubbles have proven they can change their lives—and do. A stone-cold killer such as Marlo, however, has often devolved too far into the world of violence to do anything but sneer at the idea of change. These are not smug statements of morality but of scientific fact. Groundbreaking studies done during the thirteen years I was Baltimore's health commissioner by researchers at the Johns Hopkins University, the University of Maryland, Baltimore, and Morgan State University analyzed the progress of addicts in drug treatment programs and showed that an overwhelming percentage ended their addiction and returned to useful lives (see chapter 5 for more on this topic). Meanwhile researchers such as D. P. Farrington of the Institute of Criminology at the University of Cambridge have continually shown that violence perpetrated by a youth or adolescent is a clear predictor of a continuation of violence by that person as an adult.

This is why I advocate placing nonviolent drug offenders in proven drug treatment programs rather than wasting their lives and taxpayer money on useless prison sentences. But at the same time, I believe that repeat or particularly callous violent offenders should be imprisoned until at least their mid-fifties, when experience shows that most career criminals' antisocial violent behavior significantly wanes.

By the way, as long as we're looking at that scene with the radiator, let's examine Johnny and Bubbles's actual cash needs. There are an estimated fifty-five thousand addicts in Baltimore, each with an average daily habit of about $50. That's an estimated $2.75 million a day spent on illegal drugs in Baltimore. Over the course of a year that comes to nearly $1 billion. If you are generous and say that in Baltimore City half of those addicts get that money from legal sources—from savings, family, wages, and other legitimate avenues—you are still left with a segment of the population that desperately needs about $500 million a year.

Baltimore police figure that a fencer of stolen goods will get only about $1 for every $6 in value. That means that addicts must come up with close to $3 billion in illegally obtained and fenced property to purchase drugs each year. Without any doubt, they will get it but usually from anything from purse snatching to prostitution to burglary, robbery, and murder. In Baltimore 85 to 90 percent of all felonies and misdemeanors are related to drug abuse. Not only is the drug trade the overwhelming source of crime in Baltimore, but, because so much money is involved, criminal organizations must set up sophisticated money

GIVEN A CHANCE AT REHABILITATION, NONVIOLENT ADDICTS LIKE BUBBLES HAVE PROVEN THEY CAN CHANGE THEIR LIVES—AND DO

laundering schemes to disguise it. Thus drug money slipped into the consumer stream becomes a major driver of the local economy. The more money at stake, the more likely violence or the threat of it is employed to keep things running smoothly.

IN HIS BOOK, *THE WIRE: TRUTH BE TOLD,* Rafael Alvarez—a former *Sun* reporter and script writer for the HBO series—notes that the character named Bubbles was modeled on a Baltimore heroin addict of that name. While David Simon, the creator of *The Wire*, was working as a police reporter at the Baltimore *Sun*, he was introduced to the real-life Bubbles by a city detective named Ed Burns. The two later teamed up to create *The Corner* and *The Wire*. Bubbles was a legendary informant for Burns and the city police, according to Alvarez. He died in 1992. Many of the actions attributed to the fictional version of Bubbles in *The Wire* are based on real events that the late addict shared with Simon.

But perhaps the most common reality shared by the fictional and non-fictional versions of Bubbles was his drug addiction and his drug of choice. Addicts can find crack and powder cocaine in Baltimore, and they can find marijuana, methamphetamines, morphine, and codeine. But going back at least as far as the end of World War II, Baltimore has been and remains a predominantly heroin city.

I didn't know any of this until 1987. That's the year I came to Maryland along a circuitous path that led from my boyhood home in West Los Angeles, California, to Harvard University in Cambridge, Massachusetts, and then to Emory Medical School in Atlanta. The idea of a doctor serving whole populations instead of treating individual patients was absent from my mind. I would soon discover, however, that public health was exactly what I'd been preparing myself for since the age of eight.

I grew up in Los Angeles, but actually spent about half my childhood in what was then small-town Sacramento, the state capital. That's because my dad, Tony Beilenson, was a state legislator who represented our district. Later, he represented parts of Los Angeles for twenty years in Congress. My father hailed originally from Mount Vernon, New York, and after graduating from Harvard law school hitchhiked across the country and started working as an attorney in Los Angeles. He got involved in politics and was elected at twenty-nine to the state legislature. Early in his political career, he met my mother, who was also very involved in political activities.

In the California legislature, my dad headed the state senate health and welfare committee, which became his area of expertise. As a teen, I worked in his office in Sacramento, answering letters to his constituents and writing a few to the editors of local newspapers. I learned a great deal about the legislative process and found politics fascinating. I became convinced that public service was a noble calling.

In the meantime, there was a big kid who lived next door to us named Doug Howe. He was an athletic fourteen-year-old whom I looked up to as a big brother. He was very down to earth and didn't mind taking time to play Whiffle ball with an eight-year-old kid. I thought the world of him. But in July of 1968, Doug was diagnosed with acute lymphocytic leukemia.

It's the type of cancer that today is usually curable, with a 95 percent remission rate. Back then, there was no cure, no treatment. Six weeks after his diagnosis, on September 10, Doug died. Until that summer, I had never known anyone who had died, let alone a close friend next door. I was traumatized by his death and remember very clearly telling my parents that I wanted to become a doctor.

My parents were very supportive and never belittled my earnest and perhaps naïve goal of going into medicine to help people like Doug. (In fact, the only person who ever belittled that motivation was a doctor at a prominent medical school who told me that wanting to become a doctor because a friend had died of cancer wasn't a very good reason at all.)

From that point on my dad started cutting out articles for me on all aspects of medicine, from the *New York Times*, the *Los Angeles Times*, and the *Sacramento Bee*—papers he read thoroughly every day. He did it through grade school, high school, college, and medical school. He does it to this day.

I was very focused on my goal and never changed my mind. I learned and taught CPR as a teenager and worked as a volunteer in hospital labs, and every thought—save those flights of fancy about becoming a professional baseball player—went to medicine. And so, many years later, after graduating from Harvard and from Emory Medical School in Atlanta I found myself in Baltimore, starting a family practice residency at the University of Maryland's School of Medicine.

After my internship, I took a year off to stay home and raise my young children and had a chance to reflect on my years of clinical training. I was struck by a realization: much of what we did in medicine was to repeatedly fix up folks who had ailments directly or indirectly related to behaviors or environmental factors. We'd send them back out, only to see them again and again with the same or similar problems down the road. A patient would come in with respiratory problems due to smoking. They'd be "tuned up," so to speak, but would come back time and again for the same problem only to eventually come back with lung cancer.

I saw a similar pattern in the emergency room. Patients would come in repeatedly with a variety of conditions from knife wounds to skin infections—all direct consequences of chronic substance abuse. The common theme with all of these patients is that their underlying behavioral or environmental conditions were rarely addressed. In public health, those issues are exactly what we try to address. Thus, although we don't often see the results of our efforts with individual patients as most physicians and nurses do, when we do our job correctly we reduce morbidity (illness or injury) or mortality (death) for dozens, hundreds, or thousands of individuals.

So I began to look at other options besides family medicine. I saw a story in a magazine on preventive medicine, which was described as a meshing of medicine with public health and policy. It struck me as a perfect combination of my interests. The Johns Hopkins University Bloomberg School of Public Health, reputed to be the best in the country, was just across town. The Hopkins program offered a preventive medicine residency and a master's degree in public health. The specialty resonated with me, so I applied and was accepted.

I started in the Hopkins preventive medicine residency in July of 1989. As part of those studies, I spent six months working for John Santelli, M.D., who directed the Bureau of School Health Services for the Baltimore City Health Department. Dr. Santelli had started a system of school-based health centers in Baltimore—one of the first such systems in the country. These were full medical clinics, staffed by a nurse practitioner, a nurse, a medical assistant, and a part-time physician. Right in their own school, students could receive a whole range of health services from care for asthma to family planning counseling to physical exams and lab tests.

In 1990, while I was at Johns Hopkins, I ran for a seat in the Maryland General Assembly from the forty-third district of northeast Baltimore. Although I didn't win, I learned an awful lot about the city's neighborhoods. A year later, when I ran for a city council seat, the council redrew most of my district. I found myself in a mixed midtown district made up of a large percentage of the city's gay community and large swaths of impoverished, drug-ravaged east Baltimore. Nonplussed, I canvassed twelve thousand homes, from mansions in the tony Guilford area to crack houses in east Baltimore. A central campaign issue was my push to get the city to offer more drug treatment programs and improved education.

It was on this campaign trail that I first met Kurt Schmoke, who was then mayor of Baltimore and running for reelection to a second term. We had a brief and cordial interaction, although one that I didn't think at the time had made any great impression on him. I met Schmoke several times after that at similar candidate debates where I argued for a coherent plan to hold back the spread of AIDS.

On Election Day, in another close race, I lost by seven hundred votes out of seventy thousand cast. Even so, the experience of campaigning door-to-door in impoverished parts of east Baltimore and being exposed to conditions I had never seen before sensitized me to the importance of a variety of issues for the future.

As my Hopkins residency was ending, Dr. Santelli decided to move on.

I was named to replace him as head of the Bureau of School Health at the Baltimore City Health Department. I had been on that job only a few weeks when, almost a year to the day after losing the city council race, I got a call from Mayor Schmoke. I had not seen or talked to him since his reelection. He matter-of-factly asked me if I would be interested in being the city health commissioner.

Most big-city health commissioners in the country at that time tended to be retired physicians in their fifties or sixties. Being thirty-two at the time, with no supervisory experience and in the second month of the only real job I had held outside of medical school and training, I was surprised at his interest in me. But when I met with him to discuss it, he offered me the job on the spot and I accepted.

The job came with one catch: someone else already held it. Elias Dorsey had been running the health department as acting commissioner for about two years following the resignation of Maxie Collier, M.D. (Dr. Collier had been appointed commissioner by Schmoke's predecessor as mayor, Clarence "Du" Burns.) Because Dorsey wasn't a doctor, he was not "legally" qualified for the job under city charter.

It was a sticky situation. The city's gay community had clashed with Dorsey over what it saw as a weak response to the AIDS issue. I had just run for the city council in a district where a large percentage of the population was gay and had campaigned on the need for a better response to AIDS. Schmoke wanted a doctor and someone who could assuage the gay community.

Though not immediately apparent to me at the time, I learned a valuable lesson in agreeing to take the job. Part of me feared I was too inexperienced to do the things required of the person holding that job. But I felt then—and still do now—that even if you're not sure you're ready for a position and you're offered it, take it. The things you don't know you can learn on the job, and the opportunity may never come up again. So I took it, and became the youngest big-city health commissioner in the country at the time—and the youngest in Baltimore in close to two hundred years.

As commissioner, I became chief administrator of a rather large bureaucracy with a $225 million budget and more than 1,300 employees. The job required a significant amount of time providing oversight on both the mundane (from employee absenteeism to Internet connectivity) and the important (ensuring that a mayoral directive gets taken care of quickly or addressing an outbreak of Legionnaires' disease). I became the lead testifier before federal, state, and local legislative bodies and was the official medical officer of the city. In certain circumstances—as diverse as a non-compliant tuberculosis patient to a bioterror attack—I had the authority under the city charter to quarantine individuals, to order the police to secure certain areas, and even to draft any and all local physicians to cope with an emergency.

Indeed, there was a lot of learning on the job. I had to come up to speed on a tremendous array of medical, legal, social, and public health issues—from how to abate lead paint in houses to effective AIDS prevention measures, from the proper clinical treatment of bioterrorist agents to laws on ammunition—the list went on and on.

AT ONE TIME ONE OF THE SEVEN most populous cities in the country, Baltimore boasted a population of nearly a million in its heyday in 1950. But since then, the city's size and its industrial base has been in decline. Baltimore once was a major manufacturing center; many of those industries have since moved out, leaving service industries as the main source of employment. Unfortunately, many of the jobs in the service sector are quite low paying. This, combined with a relatively high unemployment rate, resulted in a very large impoverished population. This poverty, in turn, is associated with myriad health problems—from high rates of infant mortality, AIDS, sexually transmitted diseases, and teen pregnancy to low rates of access to health care. And, of course, there is drug addiction.

During my tenure during two different mayoral administrations, I came to understand how the changing face of public health was not simply a matter of philosophical debate among academicians. Certainly the issue of addiction in Baltimore and the violence spawned by drug dealers building their empires brought me face to face with social and environmental issues of public health that commissioners of a bygone era never had to confront. But more often than not, these newer problems did not present themselves in a tidy package marked "Warning: New Paradigm Ahead."

A perfect example of the unfolding of a seemingly simple, old-fashioned public health problem that was just the tip of a very big iceberg was my involvement in the case of the Super Pride grocery chain.

The story begins in 1970 when Charles Thurgood Burns, a successful Baltimore businessman and relative of Supreme Court Justice Thurgood Marshall, bought a bankrupt supermarket called Super Jet, at East Chase and North Patterson streets in east Baltimore. A graduate of the historically black Morgan State University where he played football, Burns renamed the store Super Pride. By the time he died in 1991, he had converted that one store into seven, the largest black-owned supermarket chain in the country with yearly revenue in excess of $40 million.

THIS POVERTY, IN TURN, IS ASSOCIATED WITH MYRIAD HEALTH PROBLEMS

One of the health department's many roles is to inspect all food establishments in the city, large and small. In 1999, one of our health inspectors temporarily closed down the Super Pride store in the Pimlico area of Baltimore for selling meat at improper temperatures and for multiple other hygiene violations. One store is not such a big issue, but a couple of weeks later when we closed another Super Pride branch for similar hygiene and food handling problems, the media had a field day with it.

It led to community concern and scattered protests about the quality of food being sold in predominantly poor, black communities. I called the CEO of Super Pride to discuss what efforts he was undertaking to avoid further problems. He told me he was doing everything possible, including hiring a quality control chief and increasing training of his employees and inspections of his stores. Fairly satisfied by his response, I then checked with our food control staff to make sure we were inspecting other supermarket chains as vigorously; that we weren't unfairly targeting Super Pride. I was assured that that was not the case.

In the ensuing weeks, I started randomly checking different Super Pride stores myself during my travels through the city. I would check for rodent infestation (by looking in free-standing displays—a common nesting site for mice), I'd ask to see meat storage areas, and I'd check to make sure frozen food was actually frozen. I did find a few problems and pointed them out to the store managers.

Unfortunately, a few weeks later a third Super Pride store was closed for the same type of violations. This time, I called the CEO into my office for an emergency meeting. I told him that this publicity had to be terrible for his business, not to mention that the violations were serious public health hazards. Finally, with great frustration, he told me his big problem: he simply could not find and keep an adequate workforce.

Grocery store work is actually rather complicated. One needs to know proper handling procedures for a variety of foods and to be aware of the need to rotate stock and of the need to remove certain products by their pull dates. The CEO told me that he could not attract enough qualified applicants for the jobs he had available. The applicants he did attract almost universally had the same problem: drug addiction. Of the thirty most recent applicants for jobs in his supermarkets, he told me, twenty-seven tested positive on their drug tests.

Shortly after, with revenues at his stores continuing a rapid decline due in large part to the publicity surrounding the three closures, Super Pride went out of business. Reasons given publicly had to do with the competitive nature of the grocery business. Although few knew it, what once had been not only the largest black-owned supermarket chain in the country but also the sole supermarket chain serving large parts of Baltimore City was yet another casualty of the city's drug epidemic.

Substance abuse affects not only the people involved in the drug culture but, in a case like Super Pride, anyone who buys something from a supermarket. Beyond hurting people it undermines the economic condition of a city like Baltimore. Businesses looking to relocate don't seriously consider our city because they are afraid they will have trouble finding a drug-free, productive workforce. This turns out to be a reasonable fear.

The Wire aptly conveys across its five seasons the utter failure of society's institutions to live up to their charge to safeguard the public and to provide basic human services. If it weren't for the telling, close-up look at the lives led by the characters on *The Wire*—from cop to drug dealer to single mother to addict to school kid to politician to murderer—and the absolute sense that these glimpses are based on life on the real streets, it would be easy to say that the key failure illustrated in this series is a lax attitude toward crime and criminals by the criminal justice system. But not when we see in so many episodes the sad likes of Johnny and Bubbles pushing their supermarket shopping cart filled with scrap steel and a cast-iron radiator—although never with groceries. And while one may argue that illegal drugs is the fault of criminals and a problem for the criminal justice system to solve, it's pretty hard to arrest your way out of a case of food poisoning.

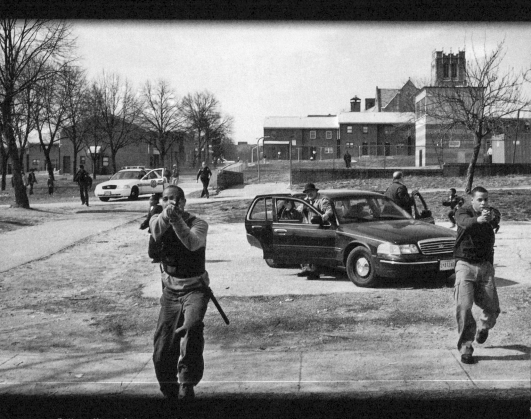

Police officers Carver and Sydnor swarm the "Pit" to arrest low level dealers and confiscate their wares, because the brass want "drugs on the table" rather than either treating addiction or going after the king-pins. Mass arrests may temporarily disrupt the action, but they do little to solve the long-term problems caused by drugs. THE WIRE/HBO ©

CHAPTER 3

LOSING THE WAR ON DRUGS

THE PIT VERSUS THE POLICE

THE BOILERPLATE STANDARD FOR MANY a Hollywood action movie is the shot just before the good guys are set to pounce hard on the camp of the bad guys. The camera zooms in on the unsuspecting tranquil world of the enemy as they ply their dirty deeds, giving viewers that one last sense of just how righteous this raid is going to be.

And so it is in Episode 3, Season 1, of *The Wire*, we see a peaceful scene just before the shock and awe of the War on Drugs comes down on what regular viewers will recognize as the Pit—the uninviting courtyard of a publicly subsidized housing project sunk deep in the bleakness of Baltimore's inner city.

Perhaps when they were brand new—unsullied by the random splotches of graffiti, boarded-up doors, and stretches of mud and weeds—these long, two-story brick apartment blocks made for a tranquil setting. For the most part during the action of the series, the courtyard is filled with young people, mostly boys, who ought to be in school. Rather, they are out there full of industry, herding together clumps of ragged drug users, both black and white, male and female, young and old. The boys doing the herding call their charges "fiends." Many fiends are bent over in pain and shuffling along where they are directed. The boys, known as "hoppers," herd their fiends into long lines that snake around the sides of one of the buildings. Here the charade begins. A big-time drug dealer does not come out and start selling the fiends some heroin in exchange for cash one by one. Rather the hoppers go down the line accepting from each fiend a small handful of cash—$20, $30, $50—which the hoppers stick into their already bulging pockets. The line inches forward, and at the end of it, another hopper places a small vial in a fiend's hands and watches that person stagger off to find a vacant house in which to crash, cook up his goods, and then begin injecting the drug into his veins.

Overseeing the routine of this daily business and unaware of what is about to unfold is twenty-one-year-old D'Angelo Barksdale. It is his uncle, Avon Barksdale, who runs the entire west Baltimore drug operation. D'Angelo is the crew boss who supervises his hoppers each day from his seat on the back of a faded orange sofa minus its cushions, as they push their vials of heroin onto a steady stream of sad-faced customers.

During a lull in the trade, two young teenage hoppers, Bodie and Wallace, sit at a chessboard balanced on a stool. But the boys don't know how to play chess, so they are using the pieces to play checkers. D'Angelo is aghast at their ignorance and proceeds to explain the game's rules.

"Game," by the way, is a term frequently used in *The Wire*. Characters on both sides of the law use it to describe either their own constant maneuverings to catch dealers in the act or to escape capture by Five-O—as the cops are known in the Pit.

D'Angelo explains the power of each of the chess pieces and the ultimate goal of knocking over the other player's king. Wallace and Bodie ask D'Angelo whether a knocked-over king is dead.

"No, the king stay the king," says D'Angelo. "Everyone stay what they is 'cept the pawns. They get capped quick."

To which Bodie replies defiantly, "Unless they some smart-ass pawns."

Meanwhile, at Baltimore police headquarters is a scene typical of *The Wire*'s take on the variable shades of gray between the good guys and the bad guys in the War on Drugs. There, Lieutenant Cedric Daniels is arguing for slowly building a solid case against Avon Barksdale that will bring down not just the drug pawns in the courtyard but also the bishops and knights and rooks and ultimately the king who runs the Pit from afar.

The cynical Ervin Burrell, deputy commissioner for operations, doesn't care about knocking off the king. He wants to look good to his superiors who want immediate arrests and publicity that will show that the mayor, facing reelection, is really fighting crime. Avon Barksdale, says Burrell, is not the issue.

"Give me three weeks of good street work," he tells Daniels. "A couple of felony warrants, a little dope on the table. That's all we need here."

Daniels and his team of detectives do not like it, fearing it will just do what drug raids always do: scoop up the low level dealers and chase away the big fish.

We now cut back to the Pit, where D'Angelo is being admonished by Wee Bey, a lieutenant in the Barksdale organization. Suddenly, an urgent cry is raised over the courtyard:

"Five-O! Five-O!"

Police cars roar into the courtyard from every direction, disgorging armed and armored cops scrambling to round up addicts and dealers fleeing in all directions. But as a squad of cops hauling a heavy battering ram heads for one of the ground level apartments, Bodie, the smart ass pawn, tells Wee Bey, "They got the wrong door. We shifted the stash yesterday."

Indeed, acting on old information, the cops find no stash of drugs and come up empty handed. As TV cameras stand by to record the typical swag of drugs and guns seized in such raids, the cops have nothing to do but cuff Bodie and D'Angelo and all of the other low level hoppers and fiends and haul them off to jail.

Those scenes underscore the core drama of *The Wire*: Bodie and D'Angelo are both pawns in what amounts to a badly played and ongoing game in the real-life farce known as the War on Drugs. But if Barksdale's minions are pawns, so too are the foot soldiers of the Baltimore police. Daniels and his special squad of narcotics detectives can do little but fume at the wrinkle this useless raid has put in their long-term strategy for making arrests that matter. For as *The Wire* aptly points out in scene after scene, the War on Drugs is all about pawns. At the end of the day, the few addicts and hoppers caught up in this dragnet will be back on the streets, back to the Pit doing what they do. The kings are still the kings while the high police brass seem just as shiny as before, as two sets of pawns go back to square one.

THOUGH FICTIONAL, THAT DRUG RAID bears enough likeness to countless real-life narcotics operations across the country in the past forty years to make a singular point: the War on Drugs as it is being waged today makes no sense at all.

The War on Drugs that the United States has been fighting in most places in the country consists of scooping up as many drug addicts and low level dealers as possible, as quickly as possible, and packing them into the criminal justice system willy-nilly. There is little effort to triage out the violent criminals from the nonviolent. In fact, the truly bad guys are left mostly alone. We seem to have washed our hands of the big traffickers who are making huge amounts of money. They use puppets to move their product up and down Interstate 95 and never have to get their hands dirty. You hear about busts but they are usually local or regional in nature. Rarely are the really top guys caught. Those guys get a free ride.

BODIE AND D'ANGELO ARE ALL PAWNS IN WHAT AMOUNTS TO A BADLY PLAYED AND ONGOING GAME IN THE REAL-LIFE FARCE KNOWN AS THE WAR ON DRUGS

Take a look at the Marlo character on *The Wire*. He's the drug kingpin who waits until the competition is knocked off—sometimes handling the matter himself or through his hired assassins Chris and Snoop—and then takes over the city's drug business. As depicted in *The Wire*, Marlo is very careful to stay at arm's length from any drug transaction. He is the type of cold-blooded murderer who should be the real focus of the criminal justice system.

Instead, the War on Drugs every year grabs thousands of addicts mostly because it's easy to do. The average addict is out searching for drugs, sometimes committing petty crimes for drug money, and is not very calculating or clever in his or her attempts. Such people are easy to find in the city's open air drug markets. Easier by a long shot than, for example, a senior at a private high school who drives to a house in the suburbs, where he buys drugs behind closed doors, then goes to a party at a friend's house where he sells his drugs—again, behind closed doors—and no one ever knows about it. Nobody sweeps down on those dealers and addicts. Cops continue to go after the easy prey just as they always have—and that is what is disturbing about our so-called War on Drugs.

This is not merely the opinion of a public health advocate. Consider the ramifications of an incident in December of 1984. An undercover Baltimore police officer named Marcellus Ward was shot and killed by drug dealers during a raid in the city by the Drug Enforcement Administration. The chaotic last moments of Ward's life were captured on the wire he was wearing. One of those who listened to that tape the following day was Kurt Schmoke, a close friend of Ward's—and the man who would one day hire me as his health commissioner.

At the time Schmoke was thirty-five and the state's attorney in Baltimore. As the city's front line prosecutor in the War on Drugs, he had been responsible for jailing hundreds of addicts and dealers. Ward's death shook him, he recalls, and he began to doubt the value of spending time, money, and lives on police stings and raids that did very little to alter the drug landscape.

Four years later, after Schmoke, a product of Harvard and Yale, became the first elected black mayor of Baltimore, he spoke before the 1988 combined meeting of the United States Conference of Mayors and the National Association of Chiefs of Police. He recently recalled that remarkable address in a conversation with Patrick McGuire.

"I rewrote the speech the night before, going back and forth on whether to raise the drug issue or not," he said. "I tried to do it in a way that I thought would spark a reasonable debate. Because what I said was we should consider the question of decriminalization of drugs. I didn't say let's legalize drugs. At the time I gave the speech I said to myself, 'Okay I'm cutting off some options here politically.' But I really did feel strongly about it, having been state's attorney and having watched what drugs were doing to the city and concluding that we couldn't prosecute and arrest our way out of the problem. And I thought it was the right forum, with the police chiefs. In fact there was another guy there, right before me, a police chief, who raised the same question. But the audience kind of smiled. And then

I came on and they suddenly paid more attention. By the time I got back to Baltimore, the Associated Press had run the story and the headlines said 'Baltimore mayor proposes legalizing drugs.' So that kind of put me on the defensive and made it far more sensational."

Schmoke's comments to the police chiefs and mayors drew an immediate invitation to appear on ABC's *Nightline* with Ted Koppel. There he repeated and expanded on his view and his change of heart from the stance he'd taken as a public prosecutor. But he began to realize that the heat of the issue had somewhat marginalized him. "By the time I got to *Nightline* it was me and the fringe against the establishment."

The fringe actually included some respected heavyweights who agreed with him. That spring, for example, Ethan Nadelman, then director of the Lindesmith Center, a drug policy research institute in New York, condemned the War on Drugs nationally in an article in *Foreign Policy*, citing courts hopelessly clogged with minor drug cases.

In the meantime, Schmoke's political future suffered. In an article in the *National Review* a few years later he wrote, "I remember the reaction in 1988 to my own call for a national debate on that war. A leading congressional liberal called me the most dangerous man in America. A national magazine referred to me as 'a nice young man who used to have a bright future.' Many of my political supporters encouraged me to drop the subject and stick to potholes."

From that point on, all an opponent had to do was reduce Schmoke's beliefs to a banal bumper sticker: "Soft on crime." Though he would be re-elected twice as mayor, Schmoke's political aspirations for higher office—governor, the U.S. Senate—were dead. He was forever more associated with the liberalization of drug laws. Now dean of the law school at Howard University in Washington, D.C., Schmoke has no regrets. "I was very committed to the issue and still am."

ONE OF THE DIFFICULT CONCEPTS for people to grasp in the Schmoke debate, both then and now, is the difference between medicalizing drugs and making drugs legal. Granted, it's a subtle distinction but nevertheless a profound one. By "medicalization," I mean we are openly addressing the drug problem and admitting that nonviolent offenders are not a danger to society but potentially to themselves. Thus, medicalizing drugs moves these nonviolent addicts into the medical system rather than the criminal justice system. It does *not* mean making drugs legal.

We tend to fund and therefore promote only the law enforcement or criminal justice approaches to the drug problem. We look to punish people rather than try to help them. Even though drug treatment programs have continually shown success at getting people to quit drugs and return to a productive life, only a small fraction of any antidrug budget of any government agency ever goes toward medical help.

America's aggressive but often short-sighted approach to its drug problem is like attempting to fix a dike that has sprung a leak. To save us all from drowning, the hole must immediately be plugged by . . . a thumb! Instead of creatively assessing the problem as perhaps one of providing dike designers and workers more help or developing new dike-building methods, we seem to do little more than shout, "Quick! We need more and bigger thumbs!"

That single-mindedness regarding America's decades-old criminal justice approach to illegal drugs comes through clearly in an excellent book by a former journalist-turned-historian, Jill Jonnes. In *Hep-Cats, Narcs and Pipe Dreams: A History of America's Romance with Illegal Drugs,* Jonnes devotes an entire chapter to the nascent drug scene in post–World War II Baltimore. Jonnes conducted interviews with some of the earliest heroin addicts in Baltimore, from 1949 on, and tracked the growing demand for heroin that started, she says, with a small, niche element of black society known as the "hipsters."

She pinpoints the hipsters' favorite territory as a section of Pennsylvania Avenue on the city's west side. Known simply as the Avenue, it attracted middle-class blacks—Baltimore was still all but segregated—and had a wide variety of clubs, night spots, and pool halls that kept the area busy. The old Royal Theater was a proud anchor of the Avenue, where audiences could see and hear stars such as Louis Armstrong, Fats Waller, Ella Fitzgerald, and Nat King Cole.

The antithesis of a hipster (a term born in the jazz age) was the "square." Hipsters wore fancy clothes and flaunted the good life to which heroin became a natural accessory. Squares toed the line. As one addict told Jonnes, "Drugs were just part of that larger lifestyle . . . to look nice, to wear a necktie and a nice shirt. I didn't come from no broken home, and the thirty or so guys who were addicts right after the war, they didn't come from no broken home either."

Hipsters, of course, needed money to buy their heroin and when they didn't have it, shoplifting became their crime of choice. According to Jonnes, the city's first drug-related shooting took place on the Avenue in 1949. "A fellow named Jimmy shot another guy at the Dreamland on Pennsylvania Avenue," a former addict told her. "Jimmy had bought this stuff and he was not satisfied with the quality of it."

To address the spread of heroin use to other parts of the city, along with an accompanying increase in larcenies, the city formed a Youth Emergency Council in 1951. Shortly thereafter a three-man police narcotics squad was formed, headed by Captain Joseph F. Carroll, a man with a fearsome reputation among drug addicts.

From there, numbers fill in the rest of the story.

In 1942, for example, according to Jonnes, seven people were arrested in connection with narcotics in Baltimore. Ten years later that figure was 242. By 1964, when heroin use had spread to neighborhoods in east and south Baltimore, police knew of a thousand addicts. By 1966 police records showed about four thousand known addicts—although a state study done in the late sixties found another 1,800 addicts in state prisons, health agencies, and the state's psychiatric register.

With an increase in the number of addicts came an increase in crime, progressing from basic theft to crimes of violence. In 1951, notes Jonnes, police records showed about 1,700 burglaries, and 402 robberies; twenty years later, she notes, burglaries stood at nearly 7,400 and robberies at nearly eleven thousand.

It was twenty years later that President Richard Nixon announced his offensive against illegal narcotics, calling it a "War on Drugs." If putting drug users in prison was the goal, it certainly succeeded. In 1980, America's prison population stood at about 300,000. By 1994, that number had grown to one million—almost one in four of them incarcerated because of possession of marijuana, according to the FBI.

Between 1980 and 2009, the adult arrest rate for drug possession or use increased by 138 percent, and the juvenile arrest rate for the same offenses increased by 33 percent. Today the United States claims the dubious record of holding more of its citizens in prison than any other country—

including China and Russia. With less than 5 percent of the world's population, the United States is home to one-quarter of all prison inmates in the world. What that means: with more than 2.3 million inmates, one in every one hundred American adults is now in jail.

To those who believe that only dangerous people are in prison, consider this unsettling fact from the Sentencing Project: More people are sent to prison in the United States for nonviolent drug offenses than for crimes of violence. Equally alarming: when we talk about "people in prison," we're really talking about people of color. One in thirty American men between the ages of twenty and thirty-four is behind bars; for black men the figure is one in nine. In Baltimore, in recent years, due to the tremendous number of arrests for nonviolent drug-related crimes, more than 50 percent of the population of black men of this age group is either in prison, in jail, or on parole!

In effect, we've criminalized an entire segment of the majority population in many cities, including Baltimore, for nonviolent crimes. In a recent book *The New Jim Crow: Mass Incarceration in an Age of Colorblindness*, civil rights advocate Michelle Alexander suggests that intentionally or not we have created a new social stratum of people who, through imprisonment, are taken out of the running for any job opportunities outside jail, have lost their right to vote and, because of their prison record will have a most difficult time finding legitimate work when and if they are released.

Since 1951 when Baltimore formed its three-man police narcotics squad, solving problems related to drug addiction has been viewed and acted on, almost without exception, in terms of arrest and punishment, rather than of prevention. Not only has that approach packed our prisons with nonviolent offenders, but also it has done nothing to slow the demand for illegal drugs, it has not reduced associated crime rates, and it certainly hasn't decreased users' demand. It's an approach that at the very least prompts the classic question, "What's wrong with this picture?"

"We need to deal with the reality of drug use and the realities of addiction in ways that minimize our reliance on coercive institutions as much as possible," says Ethan Nadelman. Blunt and impassioned about the mess we are in, Nadelman is an extraordinary crusader whom I invite each year to speak to my classes at Johns Hopkins on real-life lessons from *The Wire*. "The War on Drugs has failed to solve America's drug problem," he has said. "In fact, it bears much of the blame for drug-related crime, epidemic use of crack cocaine, and the spread of AIDS through dirty syringes."

Nadelman is one of the few people I've heard who can speak eloquently on the problem of drug abuse, not from the tired and cartoonish view of "good guys and bad guys" but from a basic understanding of the human issues that touch us all.

THE DIRECT FINANCIAL COST ALONE of imprisoning nonviolent low level users and dealers is staggering. In 2009—the most recent data year available from the federal Bureau of Justice Statistics—there were more than 2.3 million inmates in various local, state, and federal institutions. The average cost of housing each inmate, adjusted for inflation since 2001, is nearly $28,000. That's an annual expenditure of more than $44 billion. And that figure does not include any of the other criminal justice system expenses associated with the individual drug-related arrestee, such as the police, the defense attorney, the prosecutor, and court costs.

What do we get for this $28,000 investment besides keeping a nonviolent drug-addicted offender behind bars for a year? Better to look at what we don't get, which is the one thing that could help—treatment.

Only occasionally do inmates get drug treatment. Essentially, treatment services in the correctional system are an afterthought. When available, treatment is generally offered only in the last six months before an inmate is released. Meanwhile, drugs are relatively easily to find in many correctional institutions. With 85 percent of people in prison already dealing with a substance abuse problem, it's not surprising that so many addicts continue their addiction while incarcerated.

Lack of drug treatment in prison is an issue that the Human Rights Watch organization continues to criticize. In a recent report, it states: "U.S. prisons and jails remain resistant, even hostile, to evidence-based practices such as condom distribution or methadone therapy, which have proven to reduce transmission of HIV, hepatitis C, and sexually transmitted diseases and to treat drug addiction."

That's very much in line with a recent remark of Nadelman: "Police officers, generals, politicians, and guardians of public morals qualify as drug czars," he said, "but not, to date, a single doctor or public health figure. Independent commissions [with medical experts] are appointed to evaluate drug policies, only to see their recommendations ignored as politically risky."

BOTTOM LINE: TREATMENT COSTS FAR LESS THAN A JAIL CELL

Many politicians cannot or will not see the potential harm to the public's health in withholding treatment for prison inmates. Such politicians are not only acting against public health but are actually risking even greater political problems by doing nothing.

Consider the problem with HIV/AIDS.

While imprisoned, nonviolent offenders are exposed to HIV infection by either consensual or nonconsensual sexual activity (rape) that occurs regularly in correctional institutions. Already at high risk for HIV because of their drug use, these offenders are actually at higher risk "inside the walls" than out. The HIV infection rate in correctional institutions is higher than in the most-affected neighborhoods in Baltimore: close to 8 percent. In comparison, no zip code outside the walls of Baltimore has close to that rate of infection.

Undeniably, previously nonviolent addicts come out of prison in worse shape both emotionally and physically than when they entered. And they come out with a prison record, which makes it harder for them to get a job and to get out of the cycle of drug use and the drug trade.

Not only are nonviolent offenders at risk of getting AIDS in prison, but, as they are exposed to violent offenders and other sociopaths, they often become hardened or join gangs. The result is often an individual who has little chance of succeeding upon reentry to society when released from prison.

It just makes more sense to me that the $28,000 we spend annually to warehouse a nonviolent offender be shifted to long-term treatment programs that have a proven record of getting addicts back to health. Because, the raw truth is that these offenders went to prison not because they were dangerous criminals, but because they had a health problem—a *correctable* health problem—which we have for decades refused to admit to being a health problem.

The point then, for disbelievers, is to look at the bottom line: treatment costs far less than a jail cell: a methadone slot costs about $4,000 a year; intensive counseling costs about $3,000 a year; a six-month residential placement about $15,000. In a country where raising taxes is such an emotionally charged political issue, one would think that a system that saves tens of thousands of dollars of taxpayer funds *per inmate per year* would be embraced.

It is ironic that in so many states, Maryland included, the prison system is known as the Department of Corrections. What are we correcting by jamming more and more nonviolent offenders with a treatable health problem into a system incapable of correcting? We seem to forget that every day, doors of prisons open and individuals who are much more damaged and dangerous than when they entered—hardened souls whose attitudes and moral behaviors have been uncorrected to a frightening extent—walk out freely into a society that seems sadly unaware and unprepared for them.

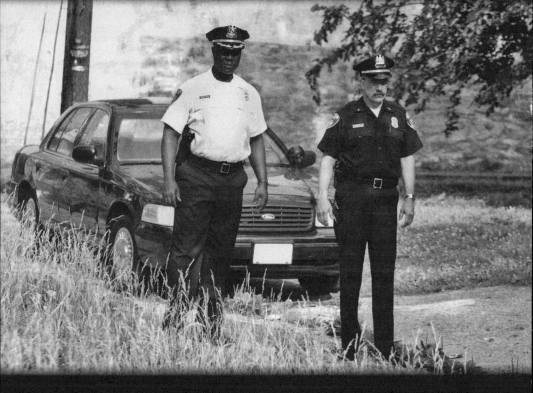

Major Colvin and Lieutenant Mello
search for a spot—later nicknamed
Hamsterdam—to make into an
arrest-free zone for the drug trade.
Unlike the Hamsterdam experiment,

CHAPTER 4

MEDICALIZE OR LEGALIZE

HAMSTERDAM

ON THE STREETS OF WEST BALTIMORE week after week for five years, a new episode of *The Wire* showed drugs being dealt and fought over with violence that was graphic, frequent, and utterly cold-blooded. Perhaps none of it was more chilling than the casual, close-up, bullet-to-the-head murders committed by Marlo Stanfield's favorite assassins, Chris and Snoop.

But there was another kind of violence depicted in *The Wire,* a bloodless form of brutality to the human spirit that I also found gut wrenching. The worst of it took place at the weekly ComStat meetings at Baltimore police headquarters. Presided over by Commissioner Ervin Burrell and his sadistic deputy, Colonel William Rawls, those sessions played out like a medieval inquisition. Police commanders were savagely berated and humiliated in front of their peers for not being able to produce or manufacture statistics, or stats, that showed crime had fallen in their districts.

In a scene during Episode 28 of Season 3, a commander is so bullied and demeaned that he becomes sick during a restroom break. Moments later as he stands before his colleagues and bosses, he is summarily fired by Burrell. When it comes the turn of Major Howard Colvin to present his stats, the man known to friends as "Bunny" admits stoically that his stats showed no drop in crime.

"Sometimes," he says, "the gods are uncooperative."

To which the commissioner viciously shoots back, "If the gods are fucking you, you find a way to fuck them back. It's Baltimore, gentlemen, the gods will not save you."

The message is clear. By hook or crook, crime stats must immediately show dramatic decreases. All of this is being done to appease Mayor Clarence Royce, whose staff demands positive drug stats as a boost to his reelection campaign.

Stung by this rebuke, Colvin returns to his district determined not to fake stats by artificially reducing felony crimes to misdemeanors—thus showing a reduction in serious crime—something shown as routine in *The Wire*. However, in a speech before a citizens' group, Colvin admits he can't promise that the crime situation will get any better.

"We can't lock up the thousands that are out on those corners," he said. "There's no place to put them if we could."

IN ATTACKING THE WAR ON DRUGS, critics use much the same argument to state their case: whether we like it or not, the flow and use of deadly drugs is a demon genie that cannot be forced back into its bottle. To spend billions each year in a forlorn hope that we can rid our world of the drug scourge is folly. But by admitting as much and committing instead to the idea of coexisting with the beast, we could begin to create useful and healthy strategies of preventing as much harm as possible.

Not long after Mayor Schmoke asked me to serve as the city's commissioner of health, I attended a speech he delivered to a community group on the topic of the War on Drugs. He talked about the tragic consequences of that failed policy and how he thought we should treat drug abuse as more of a public health problem than a criminal justice problem. However, he kept referring to this shift as decriminalizing the problem.

Because that word—decriminalization—can so easily be confused with the out and out legalizing of drugs, I was concerned that anything the mayor proposed under the guise of that term would end up politically dead in the water.

The argument that drugs should be legalized goes a step too far, in my opinion. First of all, from a basic medical standpoint it clearly is dangerous to use heroin or cocaine. Also, I believe the illegality of such drugs actually prevents a lot of people from getting involved with them. Although it may well be true that drug-related crime would be reduced if drugs were legalized, it is certainly possible that, ultimately, more people would use drugs if they were made legal and suffer the health consequences. The question: would that be better or worse for society than the decrease in crime that legalizing drugs might bring?

As much as it remains a fascinating topic for debate, the realistic bottom line is that there

COLVIN ADDED, "THIS HERE IS THE WORLD WE'VE GOT AND IT'S TIME THAT ALL OF US HAD THE GOOD SENSE TO AT LEAST ADMIT THAT MUCH"

simply is no way the United States is ever going to legalize drugs in the foreseeable future. Today that idea is clearly the "third rail" of politics (deadly to a politician's career).

I spoke with Mayor Schmoke about the issue after his speech. I told him I thought he was very courageous politically to be raising the issue, but what it really seemed like he meant was not so much decriminalizing drugs but medicalizing the drug problem. In other words, it should be cast as a public health issue, with the focus on nonviolent offenders who have a health problem, rather than a criminal justice problem. He agreed, and from then on, that was how we referred to our developing policy on drugs.

I'd actually learned the hard way about the political ramifications of even hinting at supporting nontraditional opinions regarding drugs. I was at a lacrosse game, watching my daughter play and bumped into a reporter I knew who worked for the Baltimore *Sun*. He, too, was there to watch his child playing lacrosse. In the stands we got talking about this and that and the topic moved to a new study in a few medical institutions in the United States and Canada—including one in Baltimore—that proposed to put heroin addicts in a hospital ward instead of a jail cell. I said something to the effect that I was intrigued by the concept and looked forward to what the results of the study might say. The next day's headline indicated that the city was on the verge of starting a program that would provide free heroin to drug addicts. It caused a public furor—along with my own private feeling of having been used. Mayor Schmoke, already burned by reaction to his own remarks, took me to the woodshed over my careless remark.

All of that political outrage came back like a bad dream when I watched the scenes dealing with Hamsterdam on *The Wire.* In Episode 29, Season 3, we find our fictional police major, Bunny Colvin, desperate for a way to reduce crime stats in his district. His solution is to make a deal with the drug dealers: they move off the very public corners in his district to an area of abandoned houses, sometimes called "abandominiums" or simply "the vacants." He guarantees that if they conduct their low level drug dealing there, his cops won't hassle them—as long as there is no violence. He also guarantees that if they don't, he'll harass them like they've never been harassed before.

In explaining it to the drug dealers, one cop compares the selling zone at "the vacants" to the real life experimental, soft-drug free-selling shops allowed in Amsterdam, the Netherlands. These drug dealers have never heard of Amsterdam. The name quickly becomes corrupted into Hamsterdam, a reference to the scores of addicts attracted to the area like so many hamsters.

In fact, a more analogous initiative was attempted in Zurich, Switzerland, in the late 1980s. In 1987, the Swiss government permitted drug use and sales in a part of Zurich called Platzspitz, or "Needle Park." The city characterized its approach as an enlightened effort to isolate the drug problem in an area away from residential neighborhoods, to curb AIDS, and to foster rehabilitation. However, the situation soon degenerated, as regular users of the park swelled from a few hundred at the outset in 1987 to about twenty thousand in 1992. About 25 percent of them came from other countries, and dealers from Turkey, Yugoslavia, and Lebanon moved in. Thefts and violence increased, creating anger and controversy among city residents. Some decriminalization proponents claimed that "needle park" was not actually an example of decriminalization, because it was not aimed at reducing the profit motive. That led, they argued, to dealers setting up shop in the park and selling their drugs to addicts at very high prices, thus contributing to the increase in crime. However, overwhelming opposition from a variety of fronts led to the closure of the park to the unmolested use of drugs in February 1992.

In *The Wire*, the immediate results of Bunny Colvin's Hamsterdam experiment are that crime stats indeed drop and that the citizens in his district are ecstatic to get their corners back. But when Colvin confesses to police commanders what he has done, he is accused of legalizing drugs—a major political liability for police brass and the mayor.

Once news of Hamsterdam breaks, we see a scene in the office of Mayor Royce where his political advisors are trying to come up with a positive spin on the arrest-free zones. The camera shifts to the actor cast as the commissioner of health who warns the mayor, "Be careful Clarence, if you legalize drugs they'll call you the most dangerous man in America." The actor, cast ironically by David Simon is none other than former Baltimore mayor, Kurt Schmoke.

While his successor as mayor, Martin O'Malley, was not a fan of *The Wire*, Schmoke had a different take. "I know Martin hated the show," he told Patrick McGuire in an interview. "He thought it portrayed Baltimore in such a negative light. I mean I agree with him that it didn't do for Baltimore what *Miami Vice* did for Miami, which made it look hip and cool in spite of a crime problem. Still, for what they were trying to convey—that the drug problem is a cancer that impacts a whole community—I thought *The Wire* did a good job. The characters were more three-dimensional than people had seen before in a crime drama. Consider the young boy Michael, trying his best to be good student and to protect his brother. By the end of the season, he's a hit man. That's pretty dramatic.

"But the series didn't get to an issue that I thought would change perceptions of the drug issue and that is seeing more white people affected by drugs. The series talked a little about white guys on the docks as couriers— the money part of it. But that was mostly about people warring over distribution. There's just such a huge market among whites, from teenaged to middle-aged people, that is driving this. Particularly with cocaine.

"I don't think the series conveyed that there really are two drug wars. There's the street crime guys and then there's the upper middle class far removed from the corner. I always tell people the reason we still have drug prohibition but we don't have alcohol prohibition is that folks understood alcoholism affected everybody. The alcoholic was the guy next door, your uncle, a friend. But with the drug addict, it is still us and them. If not white/ black, at least low income / upper income. You don't see the upper income in *The Wire*. They're not the ones hanging out on the corner."

Not only did Mayor Schmoke respond positively to recasting his drug strategy as one of "medicalization," he also asked me in the summer of 1994 to convene a mayor's Working Group on Drug Policy to better define our municipal approach to the problem. With his advisor, Lee Tawney, we brought together a relatively diverse group of top national drug policy experts who met in a highly structured way over the summer to come up with recommendations.

Although all members of the group were individuals who favored changes in the current national War on Drugs—which basically criminalized all drug-related behavior—the group included outright advocates for legalization, like Ethan Nadelman, as well as Patrick McCarthy, the progressive former police chief of San Jose, California.

The group came up with five main recommendations, with the first three forming a definition of what exactly we meant by medicalization:

1. Provide drug treatment on demand.

2. Reserve a portion of criminal justice funding for incarceration of violent offenders and kingpins but redirect the remainder of criminal justice funding from punishment to treatment of nonviolent drug offenders.

3. Implement harm reduction measures such as needle exchanges.

In addition, the panel recommended officially supporting research into medications that could block the effects of cocaine and launching a campaign to educate the public about the realities of the drug problem.

But the heart of the report was the three-step strategy for making medicalization a reality. The first element, treatment on demand, was a service that no government agency anywhere in the country provided but is as basic to medicalization as rushing a person with a gunshot wound to an emergency room.

Usually, when suburban addicts decide they are ready to enter some form of treatment program, they make arrangements through their own private doctors—for which insurance will likely cover much of the cost. In the case of the indigent, however, they must wait for a slot to open in one of a variety of publicly funded programs. But in the early nineties, there were far too few publicly funded drug treatment slots available to meet the need.

An addict can also enter a drug treatment program when ordered by a court. Those referrals often, but not always, take precedence over whoever else is waiting in line. The problem with court-ordered referrals is that addicts are being told they must undergo treatment, as opposed to deciding for themselves that they are ready. Does it matter? The answer is maybe, with some studies supporting coerced treatment as effective. However, there is certainly a consensus that treatment can work well when an addict is ready for it, as expressed by Lamont Coger.

He is a former addict who got clean and worked as a drug counselor in a treatment program run by the army. I met him in 1994 at a community fair he had helped to organize and was impressed with his knowledge and confidence. I hired Lamont to help run our needle exchange program— which he eventually took over as director.

"It doesn't make sense to force someone into drug treatment," he told me. "Some heroin addicts, it hasn't quite hit them. If you force it, a person might not be ready to stop being high."

He is right. In fact, for any kind of unhealthy behavior or behavior-related condition—smoking, depression, alcoholism, substance abuse, chronic overeating—people may not always be open to treatment. So you've got to have it available on demand; when people are ready for treatment is when you've got to give it to them.

It's important enough that we made it the first requirement of medicalization. We defined "on demand" as being able to provide the appropriate type of treatment within twenty-four hours of a client's voluntarily requesting it or when those who are required by the courts to enter treatment need it. The problem: it costs a lot of money to build and maintain ever-ready programs with slots always available. The bigger problem: we had very little immediate funding.

Thus, the commission proposed the second element of its medicalization definition: in order to treat addicts as people with health problems, we advocated redirecting a sizeable portion of criminal justice funds toward treatment. That meant restricting the spending of criminal justice monies to the pursuit and incarceration of violent drug-related offenders and high level traffickers—the Avon Barksdales and Marlo Stanfields of the world. Conversely, it also meant redirecting a portion of those criminal justice resources that are wasted on nonviolent offenders to a robust system of treatment on demand.

What we see far too often are the worst offenders getting deals on violent crimes such as armed robbery in exchange for testimony in another case. They may serve three years of a ten year sentence and then are released, still violent. Hence the term: revolving doors. The reason we can't keep really dangerous people in prison long enough is that we're stuffing our prisons with nonviolent offenders and making little distinction between the two. Sometimes the only way to free up more space in a prison for new inmates is to release some of the current inmates. But without a thoughtful selection strategy of keeping the violent in and letting the nonviolent out, it's inevitable that many violent offenders will be released to free up space for those who most often are nonviolent.

HIS COLD MATTER-OF-FACT RESPONSE SHOCKED ME: "CAN'T WE JUST LET THEM DIE?"

While it makes sense to move nonviolent offenders out of the criminal justice system and to treat them as individuals with a health problem that can be successfully managed, it works only if the funding freed up in the criminal justice system truly follows them. Yet, getting one bureaucracy to surrender funds to another has proven to be a very steep hill to climb.

Each of the first two points of our medicalization plan came with its own level of debate, but the commission laid down a third requirement that really stirred the fires of political controversy.

It is called "harm reduction" and is that aspect of medicalization that tacitly admits we cannot immediately break every user of his or her addiction. Basically, when individual drug users are not ready to stop using drugs, it is to the benefit of that individual and the larger community that harm reduction be employed. The needle exchange program that we put into practice in Baltimore starting in 1994 was a perfect example of this philosophy. It was designed to reduce the harm caused by injection drug use—not only to the drug user but also to the user's sex partners and offspring. The harm, of course, is contracting HIV/AIDS through intravenous drug use. Before our needle exchange program was approved, however, we had to wage a long and challenging political battle to overcome prejudices and fear. (For more on needle exchange, see chapter 5.)

Another dramatic example of harm reduction was our Narcan initiative. During Mayor O'Malley's first term in office, we found that more people in Baltimore were dying each year from drug overdoses than from homicide—and at that time the city was regularly witnessing more than three hundred murders a year. Often, out of fear of being arrested, addicts were hesitant to call for help if a partner overdosed. The tragedy is that an overdose, if treated in time, can be reversed by injection of Narcan, one of the trademark names for the drug naloxone. When injected, it very quickly reverses the effects of a narcotic such as heroin or morphine, allowing an overdose victim to breathe normally again usually in three to five minutes or less.

With funds from the Open Society Institute, we trained hundreds of addicts in how to do CPR and to administer Narcan in the event of an overdose by their partners. Those who scored at least 80 percent on a final training exam were given a vial of Narcan under my prescription. We called the program Staying Alive, and in its first year the rate of overdose deaths fell by 12 percent—the first time in five years that the number of overdose deaths was lower than that of homicides in the city.

The city has since had hundreds of documented instances of lives saved through the program. This is deep-end harm reduction, a tremendous success—although not everyone applauds the effort. When I first described the problem of drug overdoses to a senior city hall official—before we knew the Open Society Institute would fund our initiative—his cold, matter-of-fact response shocked me: "Can't we just let them die?"

Other opponents worry that without the constant fear of an overdose, addicts are encouraged by the program to continue using heroin or morphine. One such expert was Michael W. Gimbel, a former heroin addict who now directs the substance abuse program at the Sheppard Pratt Behavioral Health System in Baltimore County. He told the Baltimore *Sun* that giving Narcan "is not the best way to get addicts clean and sober and back into society." Regarding Staying Alive, he told the *Sun*, "If they're claiming that people took a class and were trained [in using Narcan], I'd love to see those people get trained in how to seek a job and go back to school. I'm still a skeptic."

Both of those comments, while common among critics, completely miss the point of harm reduction. Administering Narcan has nothing to do with getting an addict clean and sober. It has everything to do with saving a life in a given emergency. To imply it would be as easy to train someone to find a job or go back to school as to use Narcan is disingenuous. For one thing, many drug addicts already have jobs and have gone to school. Rather, our basic philosophy is that not everyone is ready for treatment at any given time. And yet these are not violent people. So to reduce harm to themselves, their sex partners, their babies, and the community because of their drug use, we believe programs like Staying Alive and a needle exchange are both humane and valuable.

One last example of harm reduction, this suggested to me by my wife, Chris Weininger. A thoughtful social worker and therapist, formerly with the privately funded Health Care for the Homeless in Baltimore, she had seen the difficulty that some of her clients have had in remaining compliant with their HIV/AIDS medications on a daily basis. (At the time, an HIV/AIDS patient typically needed to take several meds twice a day, every day.) The reasons for their lack of compliance are obvious: homeless or transient people do not generally have access to a medicine cabinet or stable location to store medicines or to an alarm clock or other timepiece to remind them when to take their meds.

In 2002, Chris suggested I adapt a program called Directly Observed Therapy (DOT) and add a unique twist. As its name implies, DOT involves having a health care worker directly observe patients as they take the appropriate medication, thus ensuring compliance with their regimen. This has been used to great effect in reducing the spread of tuberculosis among high-risk individuals in Baltimore by making sure that, with treatment, they remain noncontagious.

A similar rationale was employed with DOT for our homeless HIV/AIDS patients. The medications that are prescribed for many with HIV/AIDS reduce the viral load in a patient, resulting in longer survival as well as a decreased risk of transmitting the virus to others. Since homeless or transient HIV/AIDS patients who are also injection drug users are a group at high risk of not surviving with HIV—as well as of transmitting the virus—they are exactly the group we want to see compliant with the medications.

After some swift bureaucratic moves by my chief of staff, Dawn O'Neill, and some quickly obtained funding, we had our own DOT program up and running in just a few months. For ease of administration we tied it to our needle exchange program—since many of the clients of DOT would be needle exchange clients, as well.

In addition, our needle exchange staff were very interested in DOT. The program is actually quite cleverly constructed. Clients apply for the program at one of the needle exchange vans. If they are eligible (HIV positive and homeless or transient), they are first referred to one of two collaborating health clinics for appropriate blood work and medical assessment. If the blood work indicates the need for medication, the clinic physician calls in the prescription to one of two participating pharmacies. These pharmacies then provide a one-month boxed supply of the appropriate meds for each client and give it to our DOT / needle exchange staff. Our staff then go out twice a day to every one of our clients to observe them taking their medication.

Two years into the program, we had virtually a 100 percent compliance rate. This was critical. Partial compliance with the medications can lead to drug-resistant forms of HIV, which was already becoming a problem in certain parts of the country, including Baltimore, where up to 15 percent of new cases were resistant to HIV drugs. This could have potentially reversed all the gains of that decade and recreated an epidemic in which all AIDS cases would again have been untreatable and uniformly fatal. Yet, even with the success of these harm reduction initiatives, there are critics who would still rather see addicts locked away in prison.

"Twenty or thirty years ago," former mayor Schmoke told McGuire, "opponents would say 'Why don't these people pull themselves up by their bootstraps like I did?' Today, opponents are more likely to say, 'Why don't they pull themselves up by their bootstraps,' and then point to other African Americans who have done just that and have been successful.

"Thirty years ago there was a huge divide between what African Americans could and couldn't accomplish," said Schmoke. "Now we've got a black president. We have black Academy Award winners and corporate leaders. So the critics say 'Wait a minute. This is not our problem or the government's problem; this is an individual's problem. Why don't those individuals do what other individuals have done?' It's a big issue. Critics like Bill Bennett and James Q. Wilson articulate the values and moral side of this debate, and that's what they argue. It's a matter of an individual's personal responsibility. But the unfortunate aspect that goes counter to that argument is that the public policy of the War on Drugs has created this enormous industry that attracts people into it, and some can and some can't get work in the legitimate economy." Still, Schmoke believes that the decriminalization or medicalization debate has changed somewhat over the last twenty-plus years since he first gave his speech.

"The fundamental issue of changing national policy is still so caught up in politics and moral issues as opposed to medical science. That hasn't changed," he says. "But I think more and more people on the street understand that you can't prosecute your way out of the problem. You see some states moving toward allowing medical marijuana without much angst among their citizens. That is an indication to me that the average voter is making a distinction.

"The change is going to come from the bottom up, not the top down. We'll see it state by state. The presidents of Mexico and Colombia have talked about decriminalization at the national political level but it hasn't budged anybody in Washington. It's such a hot button issue at the national level that people would prefer to just throw money at it—give Colombia more helicopters and more guns instead of economic aid so people will stop growing this stuff."

The notion of blindly throwing more money at a problem that has had money thrown at it for decades without success should be abhorrent in American politics. In truth, it is often a cynic's way of dealing with a difficult issue while at the same time covering a political flank.

If, as Schmoke believes, change will have to come from the bottom, it means that leadership on this issue will also need to emerge at a more grassroots level. That is actually a positive thing, for it presents an opportunity for concerned individuals to not only make their voice heard but also to put forward their commonsense plans for reality-based solutions.

Public health officials can and should be a part of this organizing process, just as they have been in other crises across the years. At the end of the nineteenth century, for example, doctors were the first to issue warnings and organize citizens to action concerning dumping raw sewage into nearby rivers. Deadly cholera and typhoid fever are caused by a bacterium that contaminates a city's water source, contrary to the dozen or more quack theories popular at the time, such as "miasma," or bad air, causing disease. Doctors were also part of the solution back then, in many cases spurring the development of projects such as sand filtration systems to remove deadly bacteria from drinking water.

While the circumstances surrounding typhoid infection and drug-related gun violence are vastly different, the most basic element leading to a solution in each is as simple as Bunny Colvin's reality based wake-up call to that citizens' group on *The Wire*: "This here is the world we've got," he said, "and it's time that all of us had the good sense to at least admit that much."

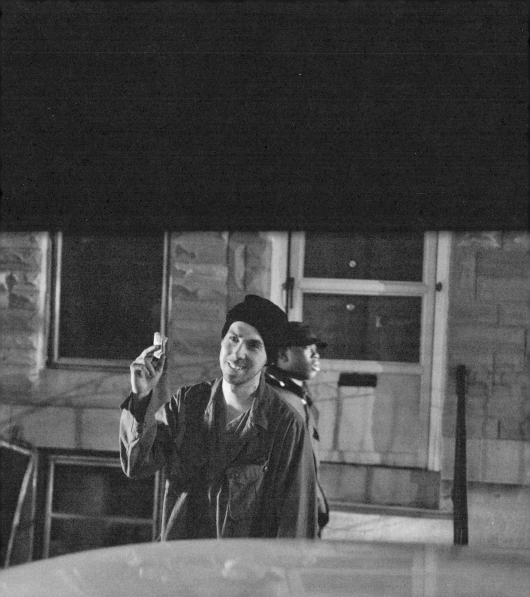

Johnny gets his daily fix of heroin. Like many drug users, he shoots up with a dirty needle and contracts AIDS. Since its inception in 1994, Baltimore's needle exchange program has dramatically reduced the incidence of "the Bug" among intravenous drug users. THE WIRE/HBO ©

CHAPTER 5

NEEDLE EXCHANGE AND THE AIDS DILEMMA

STICKING IT TO "THE BUG"

ON *THE WIRE,* AS ON THE MEAN STREETS of real life, HIV/AIDS is known as "the Bug." While it doesn't make its first appearance until almost halfway into Season 1, observant viewers will have suspected its presence from the very first episode.

That's because a used and, therefore, dirty hypodermic syringe is so often the primary delivery system for the heroin sold to desperate addicts by Avon Barksdale's teenage dealers. The same mechanism transmits the human immunodeficiency virus (HIV) into thousands of unwitting or un-caring drug seekers each year. Bubbles and Johnny—a pair of addicts on *The Wire,* who score their daily heroin fix in the courtyard of a Baltimore housing project and shoot up in nearby vacant houses—are like most of the desperate, down and out addicts seen lining up to make a buy. They do not strike a viewer as the cleanliness-next-to-Godliness type. Nor do they seem flush enough to have the money to buy a new needle every time they score some heroin.

One has to wonder: where did they get their syringes? And what happens to those needles once they've been used? Are they discarded? Shared with a friend? Or tucked away, dull but ready for the next hit? The high likelihood of a user contracting the Bug is seldom voiced and seems less important than getting their next fix. In one of the early episodes, Bubbles visits Johnny in the hospital after Johnny was severely beaten by drug dealers. Johnny tells Bubbles uneasily that the doctors say he has "the Bug." Later, the drug counselor character named Walon will quietly mention to Bubbles that he also is a carrier of the Bug.

Then, during Season 4, we see the HIV dilemma from the other side. In one of *The Wire*'s most disturbing scenes, a girl named Laetitia leaps out of her seat in Mr. Pryzbylewski's math class at Tilghman Middle School and slices her classmate Chiquan's cheek open with a blade. Blood quickly pools on the floor. Only later will a school administrator mention to Mr. Prezbo—in a revealing example of how self-preservation can trump education in an inner-city teacher's priorities—that while Chiquan needed two hundred stitches to close her wound and while her face is paralyzed and she will never be the same again—at least she was not HIV positive, meaning none of the school's employees need worry about being infected by the splattered blood.

While *The Wire* does not shrink from showing addicts injecting themselves in filthy shooting galleries or dying of overdoses, it was gratifying to see the brief scene during the Hamsterdam episodes where public health officials provided clean needles to those who flocked to police major Bunny Colvin's arrest-free zone. Still, to the higher ups in both the police department and city government, the needle exchange was just one more horrifying political blunder to overcome in the whole Hamsterdam fiasco.

I FIRST BECAME AWARE OF THE IDEA of needle exchange during my residency at Johns Hopkins in 1990 when I attended a talk by then city health commissioner, Maxie Collier. He argued forcefully that because of the problem with HIV infection in injection drug users, a needle exchange program was needed in Baltimore.

He and Mayor Schmoke had actually tried to get a needle exchange program started in the city, but political sensitivity to the issue shot the proposal down almost immediately. Yet it made great sense to me. It was a way of making it less likely that individual addicts, who would be shooting drugs anyway, would become infected with HIV. Two years later, when I was appointed as health commissioner, needle exchange was one of the first issues I tackled.

In many parts of the world, HIV/AIDS remains a huge and deadly epidemic. And even though attention to AIDS has waned in the United States since the mid-nineties, it is still a significant problem. Close to six hundred thousand people have died of AIDS in this country since the epidemic began in the 1980s, and the virus still claims more than eighteen thousand people each year, according to the Centers for Disease Control and Prevention in Atlanta (CDC). Its figures show that almost thirty-five thousand new cases of AIDS and nearly forty-three thousand new diagnoses of HIV infection were recorded in the United States in 2009, with an estimated 682,000 people now living with HIV.

Part of the waning attention is undoubtedly attributable to message fatigue. AIDS was covered heavily by the media for more than a decade after the epidemic first emerged. Another factor is the success of new drugs in fighting AIDS. As recently as the mid-nineties AIDS was the leading cause of death for American men between the ages of twenty-five and forty-four. Although still a significant cause of early mortality, the progression of an HIV infection to a diagnosis of AIDS, and the progression from diagnosis to death has been slowed markedly. Today an AIDS diagnosis is no longer uniformly fatal within a couple of years. Because it is increasingly portrayed in the media as just another chronic disease, the sense of urgency that accompanied policy and media discussions of the topic in the past has diminished.

However, the primary reason for this decreased attention also highlights the changing face of the epidemic in this country—and for that matter, around the world. What was primarily an affliction of the white homosexual population in the first decade of the epidemic has become instead a disease disproportionately affecting communities of color, poverty, and substance use.

According to the CDC, "African Americans face the most severe burden of HIV and AIDS in the nation. While blacks represent approximately 12 percent of the U.S. population, they account for almost half of people living with HIV in the United States, as well as nearly half of new infections each year." An estimated one in sixteen black men and one in thirty black women will be diagnosed with HIV annually, says the CDC.

When upper middle-class white gay men were getting sick with AIDS, they were able to mount effective advocacy campaigns to both bring attention to prejudice regarding the condition as well as the need to develop new treatments. This advocacy has declined in recent years. Many of the early advocates died of the disease a long time ago. The gay population currently living with the disease benefits from newer, more effective medications that have helped to transform AIDS to a more manageable, long-term health problem, so the urgency of their advocacy for new HIV/AIDS treatments has diminished.

Unfortunately, the safer sex prevention messages that helped decrease the incidence of new HIV infection in the gay community did not get absorbed as well by poorer, drug-using populations. Since the epidemic began in Baltimore in the mid-eighties, more AIDS diagnoses were traced to shared or dirty needles among injection drug users—whether heterosexual or homosexual—than to exclusive homosexual contact among men.

The first needle exchange program in the United States started in Tacoma, Washington. The idea came from the Netherlands, where exchanging clean for used needles was initially implemented for the purpose of halting the spread of hepatitis C. For intravenous drug use does not only spread AIDS, but hepatitis C, the most deadly form of that disease, spreads the same way.

In fact, hepatitis C is now four times more common in the United States than HIV infection and is already the leading cause of liver cancer, liver transplants, and death due to liver disease. Although a hepatitis C treatment is now available, it only attains a cure in less than two-thirds of those infected. As this is a chronic condition that often takes twenty years before serious damage occurs, the millions currently infected will be joined by millions more in the coming years, making this a truly frightening and costly epidemic. Indeed, in 2007, the Centers for Disease Control and Prevention reported that more Americans died of hepatitis C infection than from HIV infection.

As with HIV infection, the best way to prevent new infections of hepatitis C is with safer sex practices and, especially, avoiding contact with infected blood; thus, drug treatment to get injectors off of drugs, as well as needle exchanges, should help.

IN 1994 WHEN WE STARTED our needle exchange program, only a handful of places in the country had an officially sanctioned program. Congress had earlier imposed a prohibition of any federal funds being used in needle exchange programs; most public officials were very leery of the idea for fear of how it would play politically.

Today Baltimore is one of dozens of cities in the United States with a sanctioned needle exchange program. In 2009 Congress finally allowed federal funds to pay for these types of programs. Until then most legal exchange programs depended on state funding. In many states, such as Colorado, needle exchanges are still illegal, although advocates provide syringes anyway through an underground network.

In those jurisdictions where exchanges are illegal, the illegality stems from a state or local law against the possession of drug paraphernalia. That was the case in Baltimore in 1993 where starting a legally sanctioned exchange program meant getting the Maryland General Assembly to grant the city an exemption to the paraphernalia law. This was no easy task. But when I approached Mayor Schmoke about starting a needle exchange, he was more than willing to do political battle to get it passed.

"I talked about the problem being a public health problem versus a criminal justice problem," Schmoke told McGuire in an interview for this book. "So I needed some kind of public health intervention to show what public health could do."

A bill allowing Baltimore City to establish a needle exchange program by granting a dispensation from the state paraphernalia law was introduced in the General Assembly in Annapolis in 1993. Unfortunately, the bill was referred to the rather conservative Judiciary Committee, the graveyard of much progressive legislation.

This was my first legislative session as health commissioner and the first piece of legislation on which I had testified before the General Assembly. To me, the arguments for the bill made obvious sense. However, the committee chair and several of the more conservative members of the committee didn't agree, consistently stating that they felt we were simply making it easier for addicts to pursue their illegal habit. Not surprisingly, the bill was defeated in committee by a large margin.

We decided to try again the following year, and I spent several months leading up to the 1994 session laying the groundwork. Every speech I gave for the rest of 1993—on any topic whatsoever—concluded with a rationale for a needle exchange program in Baltimore and a plea to that organization to write a letter backing the legislation. This proved helpful, as I amassed several dozen endorsements from a wide variety of community groups, religious groups, and medical associations. Those endorsements got the attention of legislators during hearings on the bill in early 1994.

At the beginning of that session, Mayor Schmoke publicly declared that passage of the needle exchange bill was his legislative priority for the year—a courageous and unusual stand. In contrast, the man who had preceded Schmoke as mayor of Baltimore—William Donald Schaefer—was then governor and, though a Democrat, was very conservative on issues of drug policy. He was vociferously opposed to needle exchange, as Schmoke well remembered in his interview.

"Schaefer was so upset with the plan. He just didn't take time to appreciate what we were trying to do. Some of that was just because Schaefer and I politically weren't on the same wavelength. So he may have thought anything that I thought was good, was bad. Anytime I spoke about this, he would get red in the face. We heard that he said if we implemented this program he would have us arrested."

In fact, Mayor Schmoke and I had actually discussed forcing the governor to send state police into the city to arrest us in order to make the case for the program. Schaefer was widely admired in the state but he had a definite curmudgeonly side. As governor, he once responded to a critical letter to the editor of the Baltimore *Sun* by driving to the writer's house and confronting him as he opened his front door. So by the fall of 1993, our chances of passing the bill in the next session against Schaefer's wishes seemed unlikely.

"I spoke to so many legislators," recalls Schmoke, "but they were just waiting on a signal from Schaefer. They did not want to go against him."

In the meantime, I'd spent months lobbying Schaefer's secretary of health, Nelson Sabatini, on the importance of needle exchange. He was a respected advisor to the governor and, unbeknownst to me, had been pushing him to allow a pilot needle exchange program in Baltimore. In September of 1993, Schaefer came to Baltimore to give welcoming remarks at a conference marking the two hundredth anniversary of the Baltimore City Health Department. Normally, these would be perfunctory remarks, but the governor arrived accompanied by a large troop of news media. Secretary Sabatini winked at me as he walked past.

Schaefer's welcoming remarks soon shifted into a philosophical statement about not being an old dog who couldn't learn new tricks. He said he was willing to try new things when others didn't work, no matter how he felt about them. He concluded by saying that he didn't particularly like the idea of needle exchange but that the HIV/AIDS epidemic did not appear to be diminishing and that we should try it. Then he floored me by saying not only would he support the exemption, his administration would introduce the bill itself! Had it been any other issue, Schaefer's endorsement might have been enough to decide the case then and there. But anything involving drug policy was going to be controversial. So we carefully planned our next strategy.

In Annapolis in January of 1994 our public lobbying effort was primarily undertaken by myself and the assistant commissioner of communicable diseases, Dr. Arista Garnes. Dr. Garnes was a bright, ebullient, and energetic woman who complemented my more introverted personality very well.

We divided up the legislators and started with those from Baltimore. Armed with statistics on the number of AIDS cases in each city district of those delegates and senators, we were able to convince virtually every city legislator of the importance of the bill. But as the city delegation made up only 20 percent of the General Assembly, much lobbying remained to be done.

For the relatively few members from rural areas—Western and Southern Maryland and the Eastern Shore—most of them conservative and with virtually no one living in their districts afflicted with HIV/AIDS, we pitched our legislation as a way to save their constituents money.

It was and remains a powerful argument. With few exceptions, individuals diagnosed with HIV/AIDS due to injection drug use in Baltimore were either uninsured or on Medicaid with all costs borne by taxpayers. The average annual cost for treatment per patient at the time was about $100,000. Our needle exchange, initially to be funded solely by city dollars, would only cost a total of $165,000 to implement. Thus, preventing even two cases of HIV/AIDS would save taxpayers money. This argument worked well, particularly in the very conservative Western Maryland delegation, where more than 75 percent of the delegates voted for our bill.

Our approach to the delegations in jurisdictions surrounding Baltimore City (the mildly conservative Baltimore suburbs) was to argue that by allowing needle exchange in the city we would help curb the spread of the disease to their jurisdictions, since our borders were obviously porous. We coupled this with the $100,000 argument.

Sizing up the two major delegations from the Washington, D.C., suburbs was quite a different story. For Montgomery County's delegation, which represented one of the wealthiest and most liberal counties in the country, we made the argument that this was simply the right thing to do. It protected addicts, their partners, and their babies; it made sense.

We told them that addicts currently were picking up used syringes from the street or in some cases buying used syringes from opportunists at $2 for a bag of ten. People were also using homemade syringes. They would see a sharps container with medical waste on the street, and they'd rifle it for syringes. When you are caught up in the grips of an addiction you don't care where you get a syringe from; you just need your fix.

In Prince George's County, which has both the wealthiest African American community in the country and a significant population of impoverished drug addicted individuals—not unlike Baltimore—the approach we took was to let Baltimore do this first to see if it was something that Prince George's might eventually want to do.

Finally, for all of the legislators outside of Baltimore City we scored with an apt comment. We said essentially, "You're always complaining that the city comes to Annapolis each year begging for help and money. Well, in this case we're trying to take care of our problems and we're paying for it. All we need is an exemption from a state law."

We felt we had considerably softened up the opposition. One benefit of the governor's support of our bill was that it was automatically treated more favorably by both the House and Senate leadership. In practical terms this translated into the bill being referred to committees that were more favorable to our proposal than in years past.

Mayor Schmoke and I testified at several hearings. Because we had a sister city relationship with Rotterdam—where Schmoke had seen their needle exchange program in operation—we had the police chief from Rotterdam come over and testify. As Schmoke remarked, "This was a full court press. We wanted to show law enforcement in Europe was not opposed to this."

We were lucky to be joined in our testimony by two highly respected professionals from Johns Hopkins—Dr. John Bartlett, an internationally renowned clinical expert on AIDS, and Dr. David Vlahov, a well-known AIDS prevention researcher. Dr. Bartlett was particularly valuable, because he had briefed the legislature on HIV/AIDS issues in past sessions and was highly regarded by many of the members.

Opposition to the bill in hearings never really materialized. We fielded predictable questions about enabling addicts and sending the wrong message to kids. These were fairly easily countered by the argument that our needle exchange was only going to be serving those who would be shooting drugs anyway. It was not going to cause individuals to begin using drugs. And if our clients would be shooting drugs anyway, didn't it make sense to try to keep them from getting infected with HIV and, just as important, prevent their sex partners and babies from getting infected as well?

To reassure opponents, we promised a detailed evaluation of our pilot program by Dr. Vlahov and his colleagues at Hopkins, who would investigate our clients' drug habits, how often they exchanged needles, what their HIV status was, and whether they continued to share needles. We also allocated funding for ninety drug treatment slots to be reserved for needle exchange clients who expressed a strong interest in stopping their drug use. This alleviated the concerns of some that we were doing nothing to deal with our prospective clients' underlying drug problems.

When the bill moved to the floor of the House of Delegates, the debate became very emotional. Mayor Schmoke had done an enormous amount of behind-the-scenes lobbying and had gotten the Baltimore ministerial alliance—one of the most powerful leadership groups in the city—to finally get behind the bill.

"The ministers were starting to see a large number of funerals related to AIDS," says Schmoke, "and it was starting to get through to them that there was a problem that needed intervention."

Indeed, Elijah Cummings of Baltimore, then a delegate in the Maryland House (currently a member of Congress), was one of the first to speak. A parishioner of the New Psalmist Baptist Church in Baltimore, Cummings spoke eloquently about how AIDS was devastating his district and also about the funerals he attended weekly.

The last legislator to speak was Ruth Kirk. A delegate from east Baltimore, she had never risen before to speak on the floor of the House in her many years in office. Talking almost in a whisper, she told of her brothers who had died of AIDS because of drug use and how their promising future had been lost. When she finished, the chamber became deathly silent. The vote was called and it passed overwhelmingly, 83 to 57, a much greater margin than we would have thought possible just a month before.

We actually expected an easier path in the State Senate. The hearing process went smoothly but when it hit the Senate floor, the bill got caught unexpectedly in a political crossfire. A completely unrelated bill dealing with transportation was making its way through the Senate, strongly supported by the relatively large delegation from Montgomery County. Initially, Montgomery County's delegation thought Baltimore City was not accommodating enough of this transportation bill, so when our needle exchange bill came up for a vote, the normally very reliable and liberal Montgomery delegation voted as a bloc in opposition, defeating the bill twenty-four nays to twenty-three yeas.

Shocked, the chairman of the Economic and Environmental Affairs committee (who was a Senate sponsor of our bill) undertook a procedural maneuver that allowed for a revote. After much negotiation, one senator changed her vote and the bill squeaked by, twenty-four yeas to twenty-three nays. The governor signed the bill into law a short time later, and Baltimore City was legally allowed to run a needle exchange program.

By THE TIME OUR PROGRAM OPENED on August 12, 1994, in an unmarked Winnebago parked on North Caroline Street on Baltimore's east side, roughly 2,600 city residents had already died of AIDS and another twenty thousand had tested positive for an HIV infection. Remarkably, in selecting where to station our van, we heard no complaints from the many community groups we had asked for input. Most of them welcomed it because people close to them were either addicts or had been infected with HIV.

Our Winnebago van drew heavy media attention that first day, along with a single protester. During that first week there was scattered picketing of our site, but as people began lining up to use our services, the picketers went away. News coverage of the opening was very fair and remarkably positive. Throughout the first few days of the program, multiple stories were run or aired, with reporters repeating our assertion that this was, first and foremost, an AIDS prevention program: we were not enabling drug users, nor were we encouraging drug use.

We had envisioned attracting perhaps seven hundred people during the first three years of operations and had budgeted several thousand dollars for outreach to the drug-using community to educate them about the benefits of a needle exchange program. But before we could spend a dime, news of the program spread by word of mouth. As Lamont Coger explained, "That's pretty much how any news gets around in the drug culture."

As part of our preparation for the exchange program, we sent out counselors to talk to addicts and to prostitutes on the street. The street users were quite clear in how the program would work for them: the only way we could make a big difference was to exchange their old needles for new with someone they could trust. Thus, we decided to hire recovering addicts to staff the van. This is how our hiring panel—made up of addicts, police officers, and public health officials—found the capable Lamont Coger, among others. These recruits made all the difference, enough that we were deluged with clients from the first day and that it became clear that the advertising money could be better spent buying additional syringes. Before six months had passed, we'd enrolled seven hundred people and by the end of those first three years, we'd topped three thousand.

The program itself—which I am happy to report continues in the city today—is fairly simple. Injection drug users come to the van, where they register with a unique identifier composed of their mother's maiden name, their gender and race, and the last four digits of their Social Security number. This way they can be tracked for evaluation purposes but do not have to give their actual name if they prefer not to.

The minimum age requirement for participation in the exchange is eighteen, but the largest group of clients usually falls between thirty-seven and forty-one. On their initial visit, each client is given a yellow participation card that exempts them from the paraphernalia law. They are warned clearly and often that the card does not mean they can carry drugs.

Though set up to serve Baltimore's city residents, we have also enrolled county residents. But because the surrounding counties do not have an exemption from the paraphernalia law, the needle exchange participation cards are not legal there, and those carrying syringes without a prescription in the counties can face arrest.

THE NEEDLE EXCHANGE VAN WAS THE ONLY PLACE THAT MANY ADDICTS FELT THEY WERE BEING TREATED LIKE HUMAN BEINGS

Most city police responded well to the program from the beginning. In preparation, I attended roll calls at various districts and explained the rationale. We did have a few rogue cops taking needles away from clients and crushing the needles, stepping on them, or throwing them in the sewers. To counter this, we explained that they were at risk of cutting themselves when they handled or stepped on needles. And throwing syringes down sewer drains only means that when the needles finally do surface somewhere, somebody else will be at risk.

On a client's first visit to the van, if no syringes are brought to exchange, the client is given a "starter pack" of two syringes, condoms, gauze, and a bottle of distilled water. That's to keep them from using tap water or, worse, water from toilets in vacant houses to mix with the drug when preparing to shoot it. We provide a sterile aluminum cap to serve as a utensil in which to heat the powdered heroin with water. We give them cotton pellets to keep them from the common practice of using discarded cigarette filters to draw the heroin mixture into the syringe. Using an improper filter can cause endocarditis, a serious infection of the heart valves. We also give them alcohol wipes. If they haven't bathed—which is likely—then injecting into the skin would take in any germs on the skin, potentially leading to significant infections.

In many instances we found we were promoting healthy behavior our clients had never heard of. These are all little things but they showed that we cared. Indeed, for many addicts in Baltimore, the needle exchange van was the only place they felt they were treated as human beings. This was brought home to me one day during the Christmas season of 2004. On one of my visits to the needle exchange van, a grizzled forty-something client climbed in, seemingly to get out of the bitter cold and exchange some syringes. But when he reached into a paper bag, he pulled out what appeared to be some newspaper clippings. In fact, they were coupons for free food at McDonald's. He made a point of thanking each member of the needle exchange staff and me with a coupon, saying he was sorry he couldn't afford a better gift, but that this was his way of saying "thank you for making me feel cared for as a person." It was such a powerful statement that the memory of it still brings tears to my eyes.

After an initial visit, clients are given the same number of syringes they brought in to exchange. In addition to exchanging syringes, clients are counseled on safer shooting practices and safer sex practices and are offered HIV and tuberculosis (TB) testing.

For those who want drug treatment to get off of drugs, we initially created ninety drug treatment slots dedicated to needle exchange clients. This has since grown to almost four hundred. They filled up very quickly, but the retention rates of those early participants in drug treatment programs were relatively poor. Our needle exchange staff soon became proficient at screening those who seemed to be truly ready for treatment and started being more selective in their referrals, which has led to a much higher retention rate in treatment.

As promised to the General Assembly, the Hopkins researchers led by Dr. Vlahov conducted all the evaluations of our needle exchange program. They studied everything from the relative concentration of dirty needles near the exchange sites compared with streets far away from a needle exchange site. (The streets nearest to needle exchange sites were less sullied by used needles.) They also investigated whether the needle exchange site is a useful one at which to provide TB tests for difficult-to-reach high-risk individuals (it is).

Almost all of their studies have been published in respected national and international journals, making Baltimore's program one of the most, if not *the* most, studied needle exchange program in the world. But the key question the researchers were able to answer was the one considered to be the public health "gold standard" by which the entire program was to be judged: did participating in the needle exchange program reduce the likelihood of an injection drug user becoming infected with HIV?

It did. For all participants, the decrease in incidence (new infections) of HIV among our clients compared with a carefully selected control group of addicts not using needle exchange was about 40 percent. Among our regular clients—those who came, on average, every two weeks—the decrease in HIV was 70 percent. And, for the first one hundred or so perfect users (every syringe they got, they returned—which we were able to track because all syringes in the first three years of the program were barcoded), the HIV incidence was actually zero. Later studies of the needle exchange program showed even more significant protective effects for those who enrolled in the program.

Armed with this and other validating data, including our drug treatment placement and retention numbers, we returned to the General Assembly in 1997 to remove the "pilot" designation from our needle exchange program. This time, we encountered virtually no opposition, thanks to our annual reports to the legislature on the success of the program. When Governor Parris Glendening signed the bill into law in May, Baltimore City had a permanent exemption from the state paraphernalia law for the purpose of running a needle exchange program.

Also, thanks to the overwhelming evidence that our program was succeeding as a valuable HIV prevention tool, the State AIDS Administration took over much of the funding of the program. This funding has increased over time to the point that by 2011 the program had expanded to eleven staff members in two RVs going to eight sites around the city serving more than fourteen thousand clients. Needle exchange has been so successful that the leading cause of new HIV infection is no longer injection-drug users but heterosexual transmission.

In 1997 I appeared as the only witness for the Democratic minority at a congressional hearing on the question of federal funding for needle exchange. That year, with the House of Representatives in the hands of fairly conservative Republicans, the likelihood of congressional approval of federal funding for needle exchange seemed to be nil. However, a hearing was held by then subcommittee chairman Dennis Hastert, who would become Speaker of the House in just a couple of years. He and Representative Ernie Istook, a very conservative member from Oklahoma, were clearly opposed to needle exchange on many levels, not the least of which for personal, moral reasons.

After learning how well our program worked, however, Chairman Hastert, at the end of the hearing, said, "If all programs were as well run as Baltimore's, I would strongly consider funding such programs—except for the fact that I think needle exchange sends the wrong message to kids and therefore encourages them to use drugs. For that reason, I just can't support these programs."

Disturbed by this latest criticism of needle exchange—an intervention scientifically proven time and again to work, yet continually stymied by politics—I vowed to be able to answer this totally unproven claim. As soon as I returned to Baltimore, I called Dr. Vlahov to ask him if anyone had actually studied kids' attitudes toward needle exchange and drug use. He said no one had, but he'd like to.

Within a few months his staff had developed a survey that we helped to administer in four high schools. The study was quickly analyzed, and the bottom line was that needle exchange conclusively did not influence kids to use drugs. Thus was another political argument against needle exchange debunked.

However, this still didn't lead to federal funding for needle exchange. Again, this was 1997, nine years into the congressional ban. It was a particularly contentious time between the Republican controlled Congress and the Democratic president, Bill Clinton. The president could have exercised his authority to unilaterally release federal funding for needle exchange programs. But he too caved in to the politics of the issue, feeling he would be seen as "soft" on drugs. By 2009, with Congress and the presidency controlled by the Democrats, federal funds finally became available, allowing for the expansion of needle exchange programs in many areas of the country. Incredibly, this life-saving move was overturned just two years later, when the Republican majority in the House—using tired, disproven rhetoric, that exchanges "condone and promote drug use"— was successful in including a new ban on federal funding for needle exchanges in an omnibus spending bill. The more things change, the more they stay the same!

Bubbles struggles to stay clean by attending NA meetings, led by his sponsor, Walon. The impulse to quit using drugs can evaporate quickly if a person encounters any obstacles. Having treatment available to people when they need it is a significant factor in kicking the habit. THE WIRE/HBO ©

CHAPTER 6

TREATMENT ON DEMAND AS A STRATEGY

WALON'S SUCCESS STORY

SOMEWHERE INTO THE FIRST SEASON of *The Wire*—maybe even during Episode 1—a viewer begins to realize that this is not a show about cops and robbers even though cops and robbers seem to be everywhere. By the time the sixtieth episode has concluded at the end of Season 5, it's pretty clear that beneath all the violence and the cynicism, the writers of *The Wire* were aiming at something much more substantive than a crime drama. *The Wire* is actually a detailed answer to the question, "What happens when public institutions—the police, city government, the public school system, the newspapers—cannot live up to their stated missions of service, protection, and the seeking of truth?" The answer is shown to us through close-ups of fictional individuals whose lives are disrupted, damaged, and often destroyed by the very institutions set up to help them. The ultimate message: the characters may be played by actors, but the failures of the institutions and the terrible consequences appear as themselves.

One of those failures—the inability of our institutions to solve the riddle of drug abuse—is portrayed on many levels, from politically motivated police raids to the violence of the drug world and to the self-serving motives of politicians. But, for me, the stories of three relatively minor characters illustrate perfectly both the primary problem and its solution. Two of those characters are the oft-mentioned Bubbles and Johnny—who are the faces of everyday, street-level drug addiction. The third is Walon (portrayed by the singer-songwriter Steve Earle, who also performed some of the music for *The Wire*). Walon is a rehabilitated drug addict who leads a 12-step program in the inner city. He has had mixed success inducing Bubbles to attend meetings and to share his story with other addicts. Working against Bubbles is his friend Johnny who wants nothing to do with getting clean and who has, in fact, walked out of a treatment program and right back into drugs.

FOR USERS LIKE BUBBLES AND JOHNNY, THE ISSUE ISN'T THEIR CRIMINALITY BUT THEIR ADDICTION

Even so, toward the end of *The Wire*'s third season, Bubbles comes close to breaking free from the heroin monkey on his back. Encouraged by Walon, Bubbles stays off heroin for three days. His moment has come; he is now ready to quit. But when he tells Detective Kima Greggs he has been clean for three days and needs $200 to get some new clothes and a place to stay, her reaction is one of dismay. Not because of the $200 but because, as she says, what good is a confidential drug informant who is clean?

She ends up promising Bubs she will get him the money the next day but, in the meantime, asks him to keep informing on the Barksdale gang. Greggs, however, is shot and nearly killed that night, something Bubs doesn't learn until later. In the meantime, he waits in desperation the next day for Greggs to appear. When she doesn't, Bubs becomes discouraged. By the time McNulty conveys to Bubs that Greggs hasn't forgotten the $200, it's too late. His fragile moment has shattered, and he is back on heroin.

The truth of that sequence resonates loudly with anyone familiar with the difficulties of not only getting someone off drugs but also of getting help precisely when he or she needs it.

At the end of Season 3, when police brass crack down on Bunny Colvin's arrest-free-zone experiment, the commissioner orders a very public raid of the Hamsterdam area. During their sweep of the streets and corners and vacant buildings, they come across a body. An overdose victim. It's Johnny.

At that point in the series, viewers have been shown the three distinct outcomes of drug addiction. First, you have Johnny who is young and so utterly dependent on heroin that he rejects help—a decision that leads to his death. Next you have Bubs, older than Johnny but still not willing or able to quit his addiction and seek help. Finally, there is Walon, a veteran user, once just like Bubs and Johnny. His fragile moment of awakening coincided with an opportunity for help that he accepted.

None of the three are violent characters, but each has been a two-bit criminal at one time or another in support of the habit. Walon's rehabilitation has returned a productive citizen to fighting the good fight. Johnny is gone. It is now up to Bubs to make his ultimate choice.

IN THESE SYMPATHETIC CHARACTERIZATIONS over several seasons of *The Wire*, a viewer begins to understand that the solution to the problem is not one of punishment. That's because subtly and profoundly, the problem has been redefined and refocused. For users like Bubbles and Johnny, it must be remembered, the issue isn't their criminality but their addiction. The solution to addiction is not of the simplistic "just say no" variety, or the out-of-touch fantasy that such people should "pick themselves up, dust themselves off, and start all over again."

In my view, the value of *The Wire* is that it credibly demonstrates that addicts are subject not just to the painful impact on their lives of immoral politics and of repetitive violence. They are also victims of addiction itself. The only simple fact that resonates with truth is that addiction is a disease. Therefore, the key question regarding a real solution becomes one of public health policy: how can that disease be cured or, in more practical terms, controlled to the point where more people like Walon can rebuild their damaged lives and be in a position to help and to guide those like Bubs back to health?

As we have learned in Baltimore, the answer is not just that drug treatment is available but that we are committed to providing drug treatment on demand. This raises a larger question, perhaps, among those just coming to an understanding about the nature of addiction. Does drug treatment really work, or is it merely another misguided and wasteful process of sparing the rod and spoiling the child?

In answer, I start with a definition, given by Robert Schwartz, M.D., a longtime colleague, in his address to the students in my class on "Baltimore and *The Wire*" at Johns Hopkins.

"Addiction," says Dr. Schwartz, a psychiatrist and head of the Friends Research Institute "is a compulsive use of a psychoactive drug."

The term "compulsive," he notes, is important. It separates the addict from the social drug user. An addict feels a compulsive need to use drugs. There is a loss of control, an inability to stop. Social drug users never obsess about trying to control their usage, about when to use it or where. A social drug user who doesn't want to use, at the moment, doesn't. An addict may not want to, but does so anyway, in spite of all consequences.

It's not a matter of having a weak will. Psychoactive drugs such as heroin stimulate the same areas of the brain that motivate us to drink when thirsty or to eat when hungry. In seizing control of those brain circuits, a psychoactive drug convinces an addict that his or her very survival is at stake unless drugs are consumed. That is why it's so hard not just to quit drugs but also to stay off them.

Dr. Schwartz likes to say that "no one goes to treatment unless they have somebody's footprints on their behind." It could be family, the police, the courts, the pressure of friends, a religious conversion or, most important, the individual realizing that he or she has hit bottom. A small number of people are able to spontaneously quit their drug use. Some soldiers who became heroin addicts during the Vietnam War came home and stopped using on their own. Most addicts, however, are unable to stop without help and in the midst of their drug use are often ambivalent about seeking help.

Lamont Coger, the former addict who eventually became director of our needle exchange program, remembers what finally motivated him to enter treatment.

"I definitely used heroin as a coping mechanism," he says. "I was running away from *me*. Not liking *me*. Not knowing who I was. I tried to find me through other people, people like my cousin who used drugs. I'd hang out with them and try to determine my manhood through them and what they did and how they lived. I got caught up in their grips."

Eventually, he says, he grew tired of the life.

"My grandmother worked every day until she was eighty-six years old. She used to get up every morning and go out to work, and I'd be up there lying in bed sleeping after being out high all night. That didn't set well with me. I knew this picture was crazy. The life I was living, I was raised better. I just knew I could do better than what I was doing."

Ironically, it was his cousin who heard him voice these thoughts and drove Lamont to a VA drug treatment program in Perryville, Maryland, when he was twenty-four years old. The cousin delivered him and then left. When Lamont got clean and eventually became a drug counselor, he tried to repay the favor. But his cousin had been in treatment programs before and would never stay. He eventually died of complications of AIDS.

"The reality," says Lamont, "is that not everybody is gonna stop using drugs because not everybody wants to stop using drugs. They can't handle the realities of life and the drug is how they cope with it."

People having trouble coping with life in general are often overwhelmed by the cumbersome process of navigating the bureaucracy of getting into a drug treatment program. In 1996, as momentum for our treatment on demand program was beginning to build, I started hearing horror stories about the difficulty in negotiating the bureaucracy. The reports came both from addicts and other people familiar with the multiplicity of drug programs available throughout the city.

At the time there were forty different drug treatment programs operating in Baltimore. Funding came from a variety of sources, from private to city, state, and federal budgets. Some of them were methadone clinics, some specialized in detoxification, some in behavioral modification, some in cognitive therapy. Some of them offered outpatient counseling, while others were residential, providing both long- and short-term care.

Because of the complex nature of psychoactive drugs and their effect on multiple parts of the brain, drug treatment is not a matter of a few days of getting clean and a few counseling sessions. Each individual case is different, partly because the drug being used and the length of time it has been used have much to do with how dysfunctional an addict has become in terms of life skills and the ability to perform basic human tasks.

Overcoming the effects of drug abuse is only part of the treatment process. In fact, detoxification alone isn't really considered treatment.

Statistics show that the vast majority of addicts who get clean and leave detox without any program of care or education go back to drugs. The idea behind treatment is that addiction is a chronic disease, one that will not disappear on its own. However, the disease can be controlled if addicts are shown how to transform their lives to where they can become productive members of society and continue to abstain from drugs.

So the number of programs in Baltimore wasn't the problem. But given the complexity of treatment and the need to fit the right person to the right program, the system needed to work as a *system* and not as a crazy-quilt pattern without a basic, intuitive sense of how to get in.

What I began to hear were complaints about addicts having to wait long periods of time first to get evaluated by a program and then to get admitted. Many were having difficulty understanding which program treated which drugs and which of them had openings. Worse, I had heard that many of the programs were far from user-friendly. Remember, the idea was to make treatment available at the moment an addict decided it was time to quit. Sometimes such moments in the life of an addict are fleeting. A little bit of red tape or a negative interaction with a staff member can easily discourage someone and change his or her mind about getting clean.

I'd heard enough of these complaints that I started an undercover investigation to find out just how hard it was to get into a program. I started by creating a fictional character named "Todd Jones," who was a heroin user looking to enter a treatment program. I assumed the "Todd Jones" identity and began phoning various programs. I quickly learned that, indeed, drug treatment in Baltimore was a very difficult system to crack.

Almost every one of the twenty-four programs (randomly chosen from among the forty) I contacted had a different set of criteria for entry and a different method for intake. One program, for instance, might make itself available to callers on Mondays between 10 a.m. and noon. Another would accept calls from potential enrollees only on Wednesday from 1:30 to 3 p.m. In addition, if you did manage to navigate the system and get onto a waiting list, then you needed to call at exactly the right time every week to maintain your position on the list or you were kicked off the waiting list and had to start over.

Invariably the people answering the phones seemed unsympathetic and sounded, for all the world, like typical bureaucrats. This was in the late

1990s, before cell phone use had become nearly universal. It meant that an addict had to find a pay phone and had to have change to make the call and had to remember the various intake times for each program. Most of the time, all of this waiting and missing of phone times was just so an addict could get an interview to see if he or she qualified for treatment. Many of these addicts were transients already in need of their next fix. And, many were quickly overwhelmed by the experience and gave up.

I decided that the next step was to go out and see for myself how addicts were handled at the treatment centers. So I let my beard grow, put on sweats and an old tee shirt, some glasses, and a hat, and went calling on several programs. None of the ones I went to would even let me in the door. They told me I had to call first for an appointment. I was disheartened to find that the single program run by our own health department was the one that treated "Todd Jones" the worst.

I shed my disguise and returned to the four places I'd been turned away from, introduced myself, and asked to speak to the director. Each was chagrined as I told them I expected an immediate change of procedure and attitude. Most of all, I wanted them to treat people with dignity. They all complied.

I then arranged a group meeting to convey my displeasure to the other thirty-six programs. We immediately began working to resolve the problems. Ultimately we overhauled the entire treatment system. We changed to a universal intake system and made the time for appointment calls the same for each. No one was to be kicked off any waiting list.

When I took over as commissioner, I learned that one of the many operations already in place in the health department was a very small, quasi-public corporation. We spun that off into a larger entity called Baltimore Substance Abuse System. It centralized everything about drug treatment. You called or visited to set an appointment, you were given an intake number, and a preliminary assessment was made. In other words, treatment on demand was now approaching a reality, not a confused promise. If you wanted in, you were immediately part of the program.

Of course, everything depended on there being open slots in programs and the available funding to pay for them. At the very beginning of our medicalization / treatment on demand initiative, budget constraints kept the city from immediately funding new drug treatment slots. State and federal funding, meanwhile, remained fairly stagnant for the next few years. Thus, while there were many drug treatment programs, they were small and limited in the number of slots.

The Schmoke commission recommended the medicalization policy—which received favorable attention from national and international news media—in the 1994–95 budget. But it wasn't until 1997 that the mayor could add $2 million to the budget to fund additional treatment slots. This was the first trickle of new funding to the treatment system in years, a trickle that would soon become a river thanks to extensive advocacy work. As a result we eventually were able to almost triple state funding for treatment in the city.

This additional funding allowed the city to go from treating eleven thousand addicts to twenty-five thousand. It was still short of the estimated fifty-five thousand people addicted in Baltimore, but we didn't need to have the capacity to treat all fifty-five thousand, because not everyone is ready for treatment even if it is available. Because of this fact our more realistic goal was to have enough treatment slots available to treat the thirty thousand to thirty-five thousand addicts who would be ready for treatment in any given year. By 2010, Baltimore had reached the actual point of treatment on demand, serving more than thirty thousand addicts with the appropriate type of treatment and with virtually no waiting period.

Baltimore's funding issues regarding drug treatment are a common occurrence in cities and states across the country. For instance, in 2011, the state of Illinois cut all of its funding for treatment programs, choosing to rely, instead, on federal dollars. In the meantime, fifty-five thousand people were cut off from state programs. Nationwide, nearly 21 million people in need of drug treatment did not get it, resulting in many thousands of otherwise avoidable crimes with associated expenditures of taxpayer dollars.

By 1999 in Baltimore, we finally had enough money to start officially implementing the treatment on demand leg of the medicalization policy. One of the first things we funded was a large-scale evaluation of outcomes of patients in our treatment system. I had insisted on this study—the largest of its kind in any individual city—to finally answer an oft-repeated question from Robert Embry, one of the most influential individuals in Baltimore.

A former city councilman, housing commissioner, and president of the state board of education, Embry currently heads the Abell Foundation, a prominent regional organization. As an active member of the board of Baltimore Substance Abuse Systems, the quasi-public corporation we set up to oversee and fund the city's treatment system, Embry continually prodded me about whether we knew if the treatment system was working.

The study that would answer the question would take three years. Called Steps to Success, it was conducted by researchers at the Johns Hopkins University, the University of Maryland, and

THE RESULTS WERE REMARKABLE: A 70 PERCENT REDUCTION IN HEROIN USE ONE YEAR AFTER ENTERING TREATMENT

Morgan State University—the first time those competing institutions had all teamed up. Researchers followed about a thousand clients in methadone and drug-free (non-methadone) outpatient programs from intake through treatment and for one year after entering treatment.

The study looked at all entrants into these programs, including those who failed to continue treatment. Thus, the results were not affected by selection bias, as would have been the case if it had just looked at those who successfully completed treatment. The results, released in early 2002, were remarkable: a 70 percent reduction in heroin use one year after entering treatment, a 70 percent drop in illegal income, a 40 percent drop in arrests, and a 67 percent increase in employment. Our findings were released just as the Drug Abuse Warning Network (DAWN) of the federal Substance Abuse and Mental Health Services Administration (SAMHSA) released results of a separate nationwide survey. It showed that Baltimore had recorded the largest drop of any major city in the number of drug-related emergency room visits, clearly a side benefit of our treatment programs.

Legislators, who had in years past castigated the city for doing nothing right, were almost falling all over each other to offer praise. Republicans were actually asking for more money for treatment in Baltimore than

Democrats were. In the meantime, Governor Parris N. Glendening and the legislature added $25 million to addiction treatment and proposed adding $22 million the following year. Astonishingly, Republicans wanted to spend even more: $25 million.

Typical of the Republican response was that of Del. Robert L. Flanagan of Howard County. "We think that drug treatment is part of a strong, effective crime control package," he said. "Punitive measures certainly have a role to play, but we're not being realistic if we don't have a treatment component."

A key reason our treatment programs did so well was our creation of a program called DrugStat. Its origins date to late 1999, just before the end of Kurt Schmoke's third term as mayor. The man who would succeed him, Martin O'Malley, retained me as health commissioner and asked me to investigate an unusual management program used by the New York City police department. I traveled north and was able to observe the program, called CompStat, in action.

In spite of its name, CompStat did not originate as a computer-based program. In fact, today it's known more accurately as ComStat, the first three letters standing for command, as in command accountability. ComStat, simply stated, is the way the New York City police determine their level of success or failure at fighting crime in any given section of the city at any given time.

When it was invented in the early 1990s by a New York transit officer named Jack Maple, it was called Charts of the Future. Maple essentially pushed different colored pins into mammoth maps showing the city's subway stations, each pin designating a type of crime committed at that location. On his maps, Maple kept track of every train in the system. He used crayons to indicate violent crimes such as homicide and robbery and also made notations when a case was cleared.

The chart gave transit officers a much clearer picture of exactly where and when trouble was occurring in the city's subway system, what they referred to as "the Caves." Two years after Maple hung his maps, subway crime had fallen by 27 percent. When Maple's boss, William J. Bratton, was hired as chief of the city's police department, he brought Maple and his maps with him.

The ComStat system has evolved into a computer-driven, multilayered management philosophy that measures not only where crimes are taking place but also how well police commanders are using that information to arrest criminals and prevent recurrent crimes. Crime stats logged into the police database are crunched a number of ways to give a commander the best possible understanding of where the trouble spots are for that particular week.

If you've watched *The Wire*, you will immediately understand the process. On a regular basis—once or twice a week—district commanders are called to headquarters to give a progress report on their success or lack thereof. In *The Wire*, the fictional Commissioner Ervin H. Burrell and his deputy for operations, or deputy ops, William A. Rawls, turned those sessions into a quasi-Inquisition. Their cynicism and complete lack of human kindness in the savaging of their colleagues make for breathtaking drama.

In the real world, ComStat is used to track progress and hold commanders accountable and to plan useful strategies for attacking various issues. In 1995, a year after ComStat took hold in New York, crime had fallen by 36 percent. The system has since been adopted, not just by police departments but other types of government agencies in cities throughout the country.

Seeing how the system worked in New York City convinced me that not only was it a fine idea, but that it could also work in Baltimore in the health department. We had already amassed reams of data on health patterns across the city. When I returned to Baltimore, I immediately started several stat processes in the health department including one called DrugStat.

As a new mayor, O'Malley was more than supportive. He had campaigned on a theme of improving public safety and made procuring increased drug treatment funding from the state one of the triad of issues he emphasized throughout the campaign. When elected, he kept that promise and took it a step further—he made increasing drug treatment funding his number one priority in Annapolis in each of his first few years in office.

This stance, combined with a treatment advocacy coalition we helped to form (including community groups, recovering addicts, treatment providers, and ministers), proved to be extremely influential in attaining our eventual success. In the face of all of this pressure, then governor Parris Glendening pledged the aforementioned $25 million over three years for treatment in Baltimore City. That contributed to increasing our total treatment budget in those three years from $29 million to $63 million, the largest such increase per capita of any major city in the country. Both of Maryland's U.S. senators at the time, Barbara Mikulski and Paul Sarbanes, arranged for millions more dollars for treatment in Baltimore with an ongoing line item in the federal budget.

Our DrugStat proved to be an excellent tool for holding all of our individual treatment programs accountable. DrugStat meetings were held every other Wednesday for one hour. Each of the directors of treatment programs from the four major treatment modalities (methadone, outpatient drug-free, residential, and adolescent) appeared once every other month before two key staffers and myself. A few days prior to a specific DrugStat meeting, the program directors were sent their outcome measures for that time period—outcome measures that had been defined by consensus between the program directors and us.

Those measures were actual outcomes and included retention rates, positive urinalysis rates, client employment rates, client arrest rates during treatment, and client housing improvements from admission to discharge. Programs were required to meet the benchmarks set for each outcome or provide a written explanation as to why they had not. If a program continued to miss the benchmarks, it was given a warning and fairly quickly would lose part or all of its funding if it didn't perform to standards. Consequently, six very poorly performing programs were completely defunded.

Initially, as might be expected, there was some resistance to DrugStat on the part of some treatment program directors. However, this resistance largely melted away, with most of the program directors coming to believe that the process was helpful for both the system as a whole and their individual program—in contrast to the Inquisition-like nature of *The Wire*'s version of ComStat meetings.

It was helpful to the system because we were able to show citywide improvements in treatment outcomes since DrugStat began—particularly in retention rates and in clients' being able to get a job at discharge. The system benefited immensely from the increased state funding, which we were able to obtain, in no small part because we could show legislators that we were holding our programs accountable for how taxpayer dollars were being spent.

DrugStat also proved useful for individual programs in the manner by which best practices are shared and implemented. An example: at one of our early DrugStat meetings of residential treatment programs, one of them was doing far better than the other seven at getting actual jobs for their clients at discharge. In our discussion, it was explained by this program's director, that they didn't just provide job readiness training or job skills, but they also had employers lined up. They had found a few hotels and restaurants in their neighborhood that had been willing to take a chance with one of the program's graduating clients after the program vouched for the individual's determination and drug-free status. After that client proved to be a good hire, the hotel or restaurant continued to hire clients. Soon, most of the clients of this program were becoming employed by the time they were discharged. This approach of developing direct pipelines to employers was adopted by many of the treatment programs with similar results.

OF THE THREE ASPECTS IN THE CITY'S medicalization policy, two—harm reduction and treatment on demand—seemed almost easy to accomplish compared to the challenge of the third. Getting funds shifted from criminal justice budgets into health budgets for the purpose of drug treatment simply wasn't happening, for two reasons.

First, as always, is politics. Fund shifting was, and remains, a politically unpalatable idea. A politician who might propose redirecting resources into treatment from criminal justice could almost hear the thirty second radio spot his opponent would air repeatedly or see the bumper stickers plastered everywhere emphasizing words like "soft on drugs . . . soft on crime."

The second reason was bureaucratic turf-related issues. Although it has been proven that treating nonviolent drug offenders costs far less than incarcerating them, in fact, to make this shift, one governmental entity must surrender a part of its budget to the benefit of another in the name of savings. Loss of budget can and often does equate to loss of power. Additional funds for treatment, for example, may be added to the health department budget, but only through savings (aka, a cut) in the budget of the corrections department.

Thus, there is often great resistance on the part of one agency to sacrifice its budget to increase the budget of another agency. Even so, some creative attempts have been made to address this treatment versus incarceration debate. In 1990 the district attorney of New York's Kings County started a program aimed at providing alternative sentencing for nonviolent offenders. Called the Drug Treatment Alternatives-to-Prison Program (DTAP), also known as "drug courts," it offers convicted felony offenders without a history of violence a chance to avoid prison by entering a residential drug treatment program.

The offenders are required to plead guilty to the felony they are charged with and then must stay in the treatment program for eighteen to twenty-four months. If they quit, they are brought before a judge immediately and sentenced to prison. But if they complete the treatment program, they are released and the felony charges are dismissed.

In operation for twenty years, the program has processed almost three thousand offenders. The retention rate is about three out of every four. Nine out of ten have found employment on release. According to New York State's Department of Alcoholism and Substance Abuse, more than $48 million in funds that weren't spent on incarceration have been saved in the process. Dozens of other jurisdictions around the country, including Baltimore, have implemented similar drug courts, with solid results. Indeed, in Baltimore, drug court participants who went through treatment showed significantly lower rates of criminal recidivism than those arrestees who didn't go through drug courts.

In fact, the debate over how to balance funding between voluntary and coerced treatment programs played out constructively in Maryland. A strong advocate for coerced treatment, Lieutenant Governor Kathleen Kennedy Townsend originally insisted that the majority of new funds for drug treatment budgeted by the Glendening administration go to a program of forced treatment. Twice-a-week drug tests were to be administered to twenty-five thousand people on probation or parole. Positive tests for cocaine, heroin, or marijuana would trigger a series of escalating sanctions—for a midlevel offender, for example, the first failed test would lead to two days in jail, then five, ten, thirty, forty-five and finally a return to court for parole violation.

First Mayor Schmoke and then Mayor O'Malley and I urged that coerced treatment not squeeze out voluntary programs—which seemed a real possibility were Townsend to get her way. Rather, we pressed the state to spend more on both forms of treatment, arguing that the big savings would come from keeping people out of the criminal justice system in the first place. In the end, we compromised, with Townsend and us agreeing that 35 percent of new funding go to coerced treatment through the criminal justice system and 65 percent go to voluntary treatment through the health system.

Such efforts are concrete, though fairly unusual, examples of institutions rising to the challenge of fulfilling their contract to public service. When *The Wire* depicts an institution as failing in that service, we see it played out in scenes of high drama. In reality, while the drama may not always be as high, the petty machinations of small-minded politicians and bureaucrats who can't or won't become visionary leaders are discouraging just the same.

The Wire shows the fate of the most tragic casualties in the War on Drugs: the children. Dukie's parents literally sell the clothes off his back to support their habit. Despite his intelligence and hard work, he eventually drops out of school and becomes part of the next generation of addicts. THE WIRE/HBO ©

CHAPTER 7

SCHOOL PERFORMANCE AND THE MIA PARENT

THE TRAGEDY OF DUKIE'S EDUCATION

IF ANY CHARACTER ON *THE WIRE* stands out as the Voice of Reason, it would have to be Howard "Bunny" Colvin, the police major whose district in west Baltimore is one of those caught in the street corner tug-of-war between the cops and the Avon Barksdale drug organization. Sadly, Colvin is also the Voice of Reason Who Is Ignored, although what he has to say— some of it described in chapter 4—has much to do with the underlying social message of *The Wire*.

If fictional characters could be interviewed and Colvin were to be asked what he thought of the War on Drugs, I think he would tell you that it was broken and largely unfixable. But he wouldn't say this from any political motive or personal predilection. Colvin's beef is from the perspective of a veteran police officer.

There's an apt scene in Episode 27 of Season 3 where Colvin is trying to convey his take on the War on Drugs to the officers of his district. This takes place during a roll call meeting the morning after one of Colvin's undercover officers—Kenneth Dozerman—was shot during a drug buy gone bad.

That shooting seems to have been a turning point in Colvin's view of the status quo in fighting drugs (and parallels the real-life epiphany of Kurt Schmoke discussed in chapter 3). He starts discussing a rationale that will eventually lead to his creating Hamsterdam, the abandoned zone of vacant houses where nonviolent corner hoppers can sell their drugs without fear of arrest.

Colvin talks to his officers in the roll call meeting about the drug corners, noting that, since forever, the street corner had been, essentially, "a poor man's lounge." It was common to see men on corners drinking from bottles they'd just carried out of a liquor store. It was a practice, he noted, that the police did not interfere with. When drinking in public was outlawed, however, cops were ordered to arrest those down-and-outers, wasting hours of precious police work on a crime that wasn't really hurting anyone else.

The salvation, he tells his audience, came on the day that one of those drunks bought his daily bottle at the local liquor store and had it wrapped in a paper bag. From then on, he said, everybody started hiding their bottles in paper bags. The cops knew the score, but since they saw no obvious bottle they were free to say they saw no crime and could move on to deal with real problems.

"Dozerman got shot last night trying to buy three vials," Colvin says. In a metaphor lost on most of the police officers present, he adds, "There's never been a paper bag for drugs. Until now."

Hamsterdam, as we saw in chapter 4, is his attempt to create a paper bag situation, pushing nonviolent but nuisance addicts into a controllable area out of sight from the rest of the community. But it is an effort doomed from the start. Colvin is fired after his superiors learn about the Hamsterdam experiment—which certainly cut crime statistics in his district as his superiors ordered him to do. But this isn't the end of Colvin's role in *The Wire*. The best is saved for last—or for Season 4, anyway, which deals with the city's school system.

Out of work, Colvin is hired to help a college social work professor run a research program at Tilghman Middle School in the heart of Barksdale's west Baltimore drug territory. Colvin helps Professor David Parenti recruit troubled kids into an education experiment aimed at providing closer involvement in their lives in order to help them learn. Colvin, the realist, applies his street skills calmly and the research program begins taking some baby steps.

But regular viewers of *The Wire* realize that the experiment, shown across several episodes, is, like Hamsterdam, never going to work. That is because this research project exists in a school system that seems to do everything in its power to *not* provide its students with what they need. Mr. Prezbylewski—another ex-cop, now teaching eighth grade math—finds boxes of textbooks, video equipment, and new computers in a storeroom. They've never been opened or set up in classrooms. In a teacher planning session, he is told to keep the windows in his classroom closed and the heat on, so the kids will be drowsy and less likely to cause trouble.

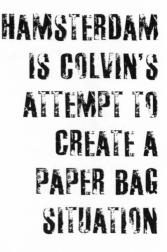

HAMSTERDAM IS COLVIN'S ATTEMPT TO CREATE A PAPER BAG SITUATION

Meanwhile, the kids themselves—the withdrawn Dukie, the sulking Michael, the loudmouth Namond, the wily Randy—most from broken homes, are either wild and uncontrollable or simply disengaged.

Predictably, school administrators eventually pull the plug on Professor Parenti's and Colvin's project. They explain that teachers must concentrate solely on showing their students how to score well on the annual statewide performance tests. If those scores are too low, the school will lose funding. Also, and obviously more importantly, jobs (their jobs) could be lost at Tilghman.

Shortly after, as Colvin and his professor friend argue at city hall for continuation of the experimental program, they are cut off in mid-sentence by a brash mayoral aide. If the schools don't teach the basic curriculum, they are told, some children will be left behind. To which an angry Colvin replies, quite reasonably, "As it is, we leave 'em *all* behind. We just don't admit it."

In depicting the failure of yet another institution of public trust, *The Wire* focuses on a handful of vulnerable eighth grade students who clearly have been left behind by the education system. In a telling scene, Bubbles tries to get his new young heroin addict friend, Sherrod—a replacement for the now dead Johnny—enrolled in Tilghman Middle School because he can't read. In a meeting with the vice principal, Sherrod is told he will start in the eighth grade. Bubbles, knowing the last grade Sherrod attended was fifth grade, objects. But the vice principal explains that the school doesn't have the resources and that it wouldn't be fair to the teachers to put an older boy in with younger kids. Thus, Sherrod is being "socially promoted" to eighth grade. Not long after, unable to keep up, he drops out.

Like Colvin and the professor, viewers of this series also become researchers, witnessing the nature of difficult young lives and understanding how the larger social failure to respond to rampant drug addiction and poverty has penetrated the once inviolate public classroom. Ironically, while Baltimore's schools are shown to be quite negatively impacted by drug abuse, it's not the students who are the abusers. In fact, public school kids in Baltimore use drugs at lower rates than either private school kids or kids from public schools in the surrounding counties.

Rather, it's the parents or family members of Baltimore's schoolchildren who are too often addicted to heroin and are so debilitated and disconnected from anything but getting more drugs. Not surprisingly, they are unable to properly parent their children.

Studies over the past decade show that more than 8 million children under eighteen lived with at least one parent who was dependent on or abused alcohol or an illicit drug. Other reports from the Substance Abuse and Mental Health Services Administration (SAMHSA), which conducts its annual National Survey on Drug Use and Health, show that in greater than 50 percent of the homes of all runaway kids, there was drug or alcohol abuse.

When parents are addicts, their children are vulnerable to physical, psychological, and emotional trauma. Given the dysfunctional behavior of addicted parents, their children are much more likely to act out their anger in public, to do poorly in school, and to show difficulties in relating normally to other kids. They are prone to depression, low self-esteem, and anxiety and attention deficit hyperactivity disorders and are likely to rebel against authority figures such as teachers. As they grow into teens and young adults, they are statistically more likely to become addicts themselves.

The Wire covers these vulnerabilities in the heartbreaking cases of characters like Duquan "Dukie" Weems, Namond Brice, and Michael Lee. Dukie's parents are addicts who sell everything they have—and everything he has, even his clothes—to buy heroin. He comes to school trailing a constant stench from wearing the same clothes day after day and not bathing. Michael Lee's mother is an addict who sells their food for drug money and spends her monthly social services check—intended to cover Michael's needs—on her drug habit. Namond's father, Raymond "Wee Bey" Brice, is serving life without parole for murders committed under Avon Barksdale's regime. Namond's witch of a mother, D'Londa, keeps brutally pushing Namond to become a drug man like his father.

DURING MY YEARS AS HEALTH COMMISSIONER, I saw many cases of children neglected because of a family drug problem. Such kids often become discouraged, drop out of school, and get roped into the drug trade. That's the lamentably realistic story of what happened to Michael Lee on *The Wire.* But while lamentable, it's also understandable. In the neighborhoods of so many of these neglected, powerless kids, the only people who seem to have money and power are the corner drug dealers.

Parental neglect is not just ignoring a child's needs in terms of food, clothing, and shelter—although all three are painfully common in these neighborhoods and certainly bad enough. Having parents who are unable or unwilling to get involved in their children's lives in a positive way is also a form of parental neglect. In reality, the kids who do make it into some of these city schools often have never been to a doctor, let alone had an opportunity to avail themselves of the basics of health services—from a physical exam to education in nutrition, sanitation, and human reproduction. In the mid-1980s, the Baltimore City Health Department began setting up school-based health centers. These are full-service clinics conveniently located in the precise spot where, up to a certain age, most of the local kids can be found each day. The man who started those clinics, among the first of their kind in the country, was my former mentor, Dr. John Santelli, now a professor at Columbia University in New York. It was he who initiated the distribution of contraceptives to students through the school-based health centers.

Having served now as the chief public health official in two areas of vastly differing socioeconomic levels, I see diametrically opposed philosophies about the need or desire for school-based health centers. In Baltimore, one of the country's poorest areas in terms of median income, there was almost a sigh of relief when we intervened. In Howard County, one of the nation's wealthiest counties, school officials don't feel it's their responsibility to monitor a child's health. School nurses there are highly resistant to having the health department come in where there isn't an urgent need for intervention, as there is in the city.

It didn't take long for me to feel that urgency in Baltimore's schools. A couple of examples:

- I was invited to speak at a student health fair at Southwestern High School. My talk was on healthy behaviors and alternatives to violence. Students in the school's junior Reserve Officer Training Corps (ROTC) were to greet me at the door and escort me inside to the fair. When I approached the front door of the school, two of the Junior ROTC boys were rolling on the ground pummeling each other. I literally had to walk over sets of legs and find my way to the site.

- During a visit to Lombard Middle School, I was just leaving the building when I heard over the loudspeakers the shrill tirade of an assistant principal castigating girls for their choice of clothes. "You girls are dressing like sluts!" was one of the comments I can't forget. Such inappropriate behavior—from an assistant principal, no less—probably would not happen in a private high school or a public school in an affluent place like Howard County.

In Howard County, my first impressions after visiting several schools was how organized and well behaved everyone seemed to be. In contrast, there is a general sense of chaos in too many of Baltimore's middle and high schools. Kids in the city live such chaotic lives that it is no wonder their lives in school are chaotic as well.

The exception, I found, was in the city's early elementary grades. I spent a lot of time as commissioner visiting kindergartens. I remember being impressed at George Street Elementary School—now demolished, but at the time, located in a neighborhood of abject poverty—by how bright eyed and eager to learn the children were. Their classroom was bright, its walls and bulletin boards cheerily decorated. The teacher was clearly eager and motivated to teach. Students answered questions and were easily as knowledgeable as were the youngsters in any of the private school kindergartens I'd visited. At that point in their lives, these children still had every potential in the world, no matter their family background.

By the time they reached fourth or fifth grade, however, I could see a remarkable change in the city children. Youngsters were now sullen, bored: there was literally a dulling of their eyes. Their social environment had caught up with them and now determined how they would behave. They seemed to have just given up. You'd see a few kids who were trying, all hunkered down. Likewise, a decent number of teachers were trying. But the lives these kids come from simply overpower whatever the school system can provide. By the time they get to middle school it's too late.

PUBLIC SCHOOL KIDS IN BALTIMORE USE DRUGS AT LOWER RATES THAN EITHER PRIVATE SCHOOL KIDS OR KIDS FROM PUBLIC SCHOOLS IN THE SURROUNDING COUNTIES

That's why Operation Safe Kids (the program mentioned in chapter 1 that led us to Corey) was a *life-saving*—not really a life-improving—program.

Part of the rationale for public health's involvement at the school level is to make sure children are as healthy as possible so that they are ready to learn and to make sure students are being treated for chronic diseases such as asthma or to ensure they get regular hearing and vision screenings. If you don't pick up a hearing or a vision problem in a four-year-old, it could easily become a long-term academic handicap.

But city schools are inundated with violence and the effects of poverty—hungry kids who are not fed at home and irritable because of that; kids often not prepared for school; or kid after kid suffering from asthma, the most common reason for school absenteeism in the city—due to flare-ups and emergency department visits. Unlike in Howard County, city of Baltimore school administrators and teachers contend with so many issues that it is understandable why they didn't push back when the health department announced it was moving in. By dealing with health issues that often affected the school environment, the health department was leaving the beleaguered school system with one fewer problem to address.

Tragically, one of the conditions most important to be addressed in school-based health centers is the issue of violence and how it affects a child. Posttraumatic stress disorder (PTSD) and depression are related issues that come up again and again. Fortunately, society has come a long way in its capacity to understand and deal with PTSD. But only in the last decade or so has a diagnosis of PTSD been viewed seriously, even in the military. It certainly has had little credibility in domestic life. But on a daily basis, children in many city schools describe violence they have witnessed or been party to.

In a city high school setting one of our mental health professionals asked a roomful of about fifty teens how many had either seen, been victims of, or had family members who were victims of violence. Almost all of them could cite one degree of separation from a violent act. They saw a friend being shot and killed or an uncle paralyzed from the waist down, and virtually all had witnessed acts of brutality resulting in injury. This repeated exposure to violence can cause an immense amount of trauma that can in turn lead to serious emotional issues. Indeed, it is the root of much of the depression that is so common among city students. To combat the endemic nature of mental health issues in the schools, each of the city's school-based health centers has psychologists and social workers to provide care to students. Treatment can include medication, cognitive behavioral therapy, and group therapy. One of the school centers started grief groups to help kids who'd experienced the violent death of someone close. These are strategies that can take the edge off of the anger and grief in a youngster's life and allow a child a chance to learn.

ALTHOUGH AN ADDICTED PARENT can become physically, or even sexually abusive to children, as was the case with the fictional Michael Lee, sometimes their prolonged absences from home while out looking for drugs can cause as much emotional distress. I saw a good example of that when I was a part-time provider at one of the school-based health centers at a middle school in the heart of drug-infested west Baltimore. Frequently I would be called in for a second opinion or when a case was particularly difficult to diagnose. One day the nurse practitioner who ran the school's health center asked me to review the case of a fourteen-year-old girl whom I'll refer to as "Maria."

She was referred to the health center by a teacher who was concerned that Maria was frequently falling asleep in class. Her teacher thought there might be something wrong with her. She was normally an A student who had never shown any problems before.

When Maria came into the exam room, I did all of the appropriate medical things one does when fatigue is the complaint. That includes an evaluation of her hematocrit—a test that measures the percentage of red blood cells, often used to diagnose anemia, a frequent cause of fatigue in teenage girls. Maria's blood work was normal, as was the rest of her physical exam. In circumstances such as this the most important thing a physician can do is to take a detailed history. As Maria began telling me about her home situation the cause of her fatigue became obvious. Quite simply, she was exhausted by her life circumstances.

It turned out that this young woman, who managed to keep up a B average despite her sleepiness, was the de facto primary caretaker in her household. Maria's father was incarcerated for a drug-related dispute. Her mom, also an addict, was in and out of the family and was currently nowhere to be found. Maria took care of her seventy-seven-year-old grandfather—who sounded like he had early Alzheimer's disease—and her five-year-old brother, whom she got to bed at night and woke up in the morning and for whom she made lunch every day. This remarkable young woman went shopping every day for her little family (in many parts of Baltimore there are no supermarkets, only small, grossly overpriced corner grocery stores) because she couldn't carry more than a day's worth of groceries back to her row house. She had to hurry home to make sure her grandfather didn't wander off, which he frequently did. The fact that she was able to do her homework and keep up her grades was what was astounding.

Maria is not alone in Baltimore. In fact, such situations are tragically common, with the usual result being children who come to school completely unable to learn or perform. Because of this, our public schools start off behind the "eight ball," a position compounded by a lack of enough truly caring teachers who might be able to step in and help. Thus, we have astoundingly high dropout rates—at most of Baltimore's high schools in the 1990s and early 2000s fewer than 30 percent of the students who entered the ninth grade went on to graduate. Those who did finish often lacked basic reading and writing skills.

That's why Kid Stat (discussed in chapter 1) was so useful. As we did with Corey and other potential murder victims, we were able to bring a tremendous amount of services to bear on kids' lives. In a less urgent situation, as in Maria's case, we had to depend on public social service agencies and assume they would follow up with their client. The trouble was that in an overwhelmed system, a case like Maria's was not a huge priority. She was not being physically or sexually abused. She was in pretty decent shape, but hers was nowhere near the kind of emergency case like Corey that demands immediate attention, and therein lies the rub.

In a perfect system—or at least a well-organized one—paying attention to problems facing young people, immediate or otherwise, is presumed to be important. To put it another way, there is at least a public expectation that government agencies will act in the public interest. Unfortunately, in certain city neighborhoods, that is a presumption that borders on fantasy. Reasonable minds might suggest that in addition to "well-organized" we insert "well-funded" in the formula.

THIS IS WHERE *THE WIRE* STEPS IN with its palpably realistic story line of uncaring, overburdened, and underfunded bureaucracies running through all five of its seasons. The effect is to remind us that not only do we live in an imperfect and often disorganized world but that public expectations are also colored by a certain degree of cynicism. Even so, cops undermining fellow cops and politicians doing dirt to other politicians pales in comparison to the visceral, spirit-robbing misery that such human failings perpetrate on children—as seen in Season 4's close-up of the school system.

In that connection, one of the difficult issues I faced in my early days as health commissioner was the extremely high rate of children in city schools who hadn't been immunized against measles, mumps, and smallpox. Two out of every five kids enrolled in public schools hadn't gotten their shots—even though state law mandated that before children could be admitted to kindergarten at the start of a school year, so they had to show proof of compliance. Not surprisingly, the majority of the children who hadn't been vaccinated came from the heart of the poorest and most drug-infested parts of the city.

At various times I had urged and even harassed the school system over their low rates of immunization, but the central administration continually dragged its feet. It puzzled me as to why the situation had been allowed to deteriorate so long. Measles, for example, can be a deadly disease, is often quite serious, and is readily contagious, yet eminently preventable with vaccinations.

Gradually, the reason for the school system's lack of cooperation dawned on me. Early each school year, in the fall, the number of students enrolled on a specific date on the school calendar determines the amount of capitated—fee per student—state aid paid to that school system. The more students enrolled on that magic date, the more state funding received. (This issue is cynically shown in *The Wire*, when Dennis "Cutty" Wise and others are paid to round up students for the beginning of the school year. Later they are told that their services are no longer needed. The time that schools are being paid per student is over for the year.) If the schools followed the law, however, they would have to turn away children not fully immunized, subtracting—at that the 1994 rate of noncompliance—40 percent of its enrollment by the capitation date.

Between 1989 and 1991 a major measles resurgence occurred in many areas of the United States, including Baltimore. The city recorded over one hundred cases in two years, part of the fifty-five thousand cases reported nationwide that claimed 123 lives and hospitalized eleven thousand. This was an unexpected jump in the number of cases; health officials across the country had previously met with success in their efforts to eliminate all measles cases in the United States.

The main cause for the resurgence was the low number of children who had been vaccinated by the age of two. In some areas of the country, as few as 50 percent of children had received their shots. A survey showed that the majority of children who didn't get their vaccinations were black and Hispanic. Yet not even that ominous warning moved the city's schools to do something about their low vaccination rate. Simply put, the school system had pushed this health concern to the back burner and had not enforced the law for many years.

The issue came to a head in an odd and embarrassing way. It started in 1994 when the Clinton administration was trying to get more congressional funding for the Agency for International Development (AID). Vice president Al Gore helped set up a program called Lessons without Borders to connect cities in the United States with AID projects overseas. The idea was to show the program's value by putting into practice in this country some of the lessons learned in so-called third world countries. Gore came to Baltimore to announce that we would be the pilot city—a bit of a sad commentary on the state of Baltimore's problems.

With the assistance of AID, and the encouragement of the vice president, we sent an assistant commissioner to Kenya to observe their immunization program, which had achieved high rates of compliance. When she returned we found we had the ammunition we needed to force the school administration's hand. Mayor Schmoke confronted the superintendent of schools with an awkward fact. "Kenya does this way better than we do," he said. "There's no excuse. You're going to have to play ball with Peter."

We decided on an aggressive course of action. First, we would enforce the law that kids who were not fully immunized would not be allowed to enter school—unless they had a slip proving they had an appointment with their pediatrician in the next twenty days to get their shots. Second, any child who was excluded from school for noncompliance and who did not return to school with the required shots or appointment slip within twenty days would be deemed a truant.

We then went to the city state's attorney (the equivalent of a district attorney in Maryland) to get her agreement to prosecute the parents of these kids on truancy charges. This, of course, was not done with the intent of going after parents and to break up families; rather, it was to make a statement about how seriously we were taking this issue.

In late August, we mounted a campaign to publicize our new policy, using all modes of media, including public service announcements and regular coverage of those messages by all local television stations. To make it easier for parents to get their kids immunized, we held mass immunization clinics at the school headquarters building, using dozens of our health department nurses and doctors. All of these efforts were very successful, reducing the number of noncompliant kids from about forty thousand to one thousand by the time school started. As soon as the parents of those thousand students saw we were serious—as evidenced by their exclusion from school—80 percent of them got their shots within a few days. Finally, to deal with the remaining two hundred or so children who ended up being deemed truant (by virtue of missing twenty days), we got the state's attorney to send letters to all of their parents threatening prosecution—though none ended up needing to be prosecuted.

By November of the 1995–96 school year we had achieved a 99.9 percent immunization compliance rate in a school system that had languished in the 60 percent range for years. By the way, in 2000, public health officials achieved their goal of eliminating measles in the United States. Since then fewer than one case per million has been reported in this country—against the high in the 1950s of 313 per 100,000.

Today the city continues to maintain a 99.8 percent immunization compliance rate in its public schools. To date the city has had virtually no cases of measles or mumps—a testament to the positive role public health can and must play in resolving health issues that are complicated by social disruption.

EVER SINCE WATCHING *THE WIRE*, I had been curious as to the take of my old boss, Kurt Schmoke, on the program's treatment of the city's schools. I knew how much time he'd put into trying to change them for the better. Coauthor Patrick McGuire caught up with the former mayor and asked him. His reply, as usual, was candid and thought provoking.

"I think *The Wire* was fair in its treatment of the schools," he said, "although what they didn't show was that there are some schools that are very successful and many teachers doing a very good job. Some schools do quite well but there are a huge number of schools in the heart of the city where poverty and drug problems just infected everything. Kids' parents would be on drugs. More than a third of our kids changed schools in the middle of the year. You can imagine how totally disruptive that is to not only them but to everybody else: people getting evicted from homes, getting arrested, and moving their kids. The drug problem had a huge impact on elementary and middle schools.

"The one thing I wanted to do most as mayor that I did not succeed in was a dramatic reform of public education. I wanted to leave office with a school system where excellence was viewed as the rule, not the exception. I left it pretty much as I found it, which was pockets of excellence, but still a lot of really serious problems. The reason for that, and something I didn't recognize coming in, was the budget of the school system. It was controlled one-third by local government, one-third by the state, and one-third by the feds. So if you were going to make major changes, all three areas of government had to be aligned. And, in fact, all three had their own views of where the schools should go. That's why it was extraordinarily difficult."

The Wire never quite lays out this sort of real world rationale for the depressing gridlock that strangled initiative and creativity from the top down in Baltimore's public education system. As this is a fictional version of Baltimore, the school system as a whole is cast as a one-dimensional heavy, indifferent to the frustrations suffocating teachers and, thus, turning off students at Tilghman Middle School to the possibility of learning something.

While Tilghman's administrators and teachers are depicted as much rounder characters with traits both noble and questionable—as is representative of the real world—the system's leadership is cold enough to pull the rug on Bunny Colvin's sociological experiment while insisting that time spent raising standardized test scores was much more important. The idea being that test scores made the administrators look good, even if the students looked like they always did: sleepy, angry, ignorant, and disconnected. Here too, in today's era of No Child Left Behind, this depiction is not completely fair, since schools—not just administrators—face significant consequences for poor test scores. I think we as a country have gone way too far in terms of rewarding "teaching to the test."

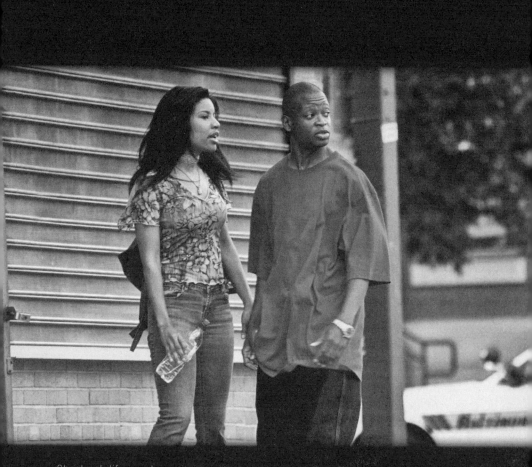

Shardene's life as a dancer in a
"gentlemen's club" put her at risk
for sexually transmitted diseases
and unwanted pregnancies. Providing birth control and testing
for STDs gives people options and
allows young women to finish
school and to escape the cycle
of poverty. THE WIRE/HBO ©

CHAPTER 8

TEENAGE PREGNANCY AND STDs

SHARDENE'S ESCAPE

A FREQUENT SCENE OF THE ACTION in the first year's episodes of *The Wire* is the fictional west Baltimore bar known as Orlando's Gentleman's Club. In spite of the fancy name, it's really no place for gentlemen and is, in fact, a stripper bar. The Orlando in the name is an employee of the Avon Barksdale drug organization. The day's proceeds from all drugs sold on street corners and in public housing complexes make their way to the second floor offices of Orlando's, where Barksdale's chief lieutenant, Russell "Stringer" Bell, glowers, counts the money, and glowers some more.

It is here that we see young D'Angelo Barksdale, Avon's nephew, who has recently been acquitted of a murder because his uncle bribed a witness. In spite of his guilt, D'Angelo doesn't seem the cold-blooded type when compared with Avon or Stringer Bell. Though D'Angelo—or Dee as he is called—has a girlfriend who is the mother of his child, we see him falling hard for one of Orlando's strippers.

Shardene Innes, however, isn't just another prostitute at Orlando's. She is quick to point out to Dee that she doesn't do drugs and she isn't a hooker as are most of the other dancers there. Still, she recognizes an opportunity when it comes her way, as D'Angelo overstates his authority, bragging about being his uncle's right hand man.

When Shardene becomes sexually involved with D'Angelo, played out in Episodes 8 and 9 of *The Wire*'s first season, she learns about his girlfriend and his eleven-month-old son. In a telling moment, where Dee seems torn between feelings of shame and the need to act the swaggering male, he demeans both Shardene and his girlfriend with a dismissive sexual insult. It's enough to trigger the disillusionment of Shardene, who has already given voice to anxieties about her uncertain future, by saying, "I can't stay pretty forever."

In the eyes of Detective Lester Freamon of the major crimes squad investigating Avon Barksdale, Shardene appears the perfect candidate to be recruited as an informant. He wins Shardene's loyalty by showing her pictures of the body of a dead stripper—a friend of hers who overdosed at a Barksdale gang party. Her body had been wrapped in a carpet and tossed into a dumpster. Later, when Dee is surprised to find Shardene clearing out of his apartment, she says, "Do I look like someone you can roll up in a rug and throw in the trash?"

While *The Wire* never directly touches on syphilis or teen pregnancy, in the character of Shardene it nevertheless strikes at the heart of those issues. In depicting the casual debasement of women, *The Wire* in Season 1 begins to connect the dots we too often pretend not to see between the abuse of power and the undermining of social order. In its five seasons, *The Wire* unequivocally exposes irresponsibility in public institutions such as the media, education, and government. In its first season, however, it reminds us that the most basic corruption is the perversion of self.

As *The Wire* graphically shows, there's plenty of perversion to go around in the culture of drug dealing and addiction. There's a revealing sequence in Season 3 where the Dennis Wise character, known as Cutty, is out of prison after a long term and is being recruited back into the game by the Barksdale gang. One night he is invited to a party filled with drugs, booze, and plenty of eager women. Everybody seems stoned and depravity reigns. Later, Cutty backs away from a return to crime when he realizes that murder as a price for staying in the game has lost its allure. His epiphany is rare.

In both the fictional backdrop of *The Wire* and the streets of everyday real life, the ultimate price paid for a drug culture lifestyle is the ruination of lives—from individuals to entire families. Unwanted pregnancies and unprotected sex with multiple partners are often the first steps in a life of misery—misery that could be if not prevented at least reduced—and *The Wire* mines this reality in several of its characters, including the young teen Michael Lee. To get money to buy drugs, his hopeless mother sells everything from food in the refrigerator to her body. As a consequence she has produced children—Michael and his younger brother nicknamed Bug—that she can't and won't care for.

Taken as a whole, these story arcs are to me more than fictional devices to move along the saga of the Barksdale gang. They are telling symptoms of the disease of addiction. Without question, the risk-filled lifestyle of the drug culture is a common link between real-world issues of teen pregnancy and sexually transmitted diseases, or STDs, such as syphilis. While public health measures taken in Baltimore and across the country have succeeded in lowering the rates of both, the connection to the drug trade and addiction continues to make each issue a continuing threat.

A BASIC STEP TOWARD FINDING SOLUTIONS to such problems is to stop kidding ourselves and admit that teenage sexuality is a natural fact of life. Studies from around the country show that about 70 percent of all high school seniors are sexually active by the time they graduate. As with many health and social trends, the socioeconomic status of the participants marks the main difference in how often irresponsible or unsafe sexual practices lead to negative consequences.

While the rate of sexual activity and the incidence of sexually transmitted diseases varies little between socioeconomic classes, it is obvious that those of greater means are much more likely to have access to comprehensive contraceptive and abortion services. In other words, the teen birth problem in this country is largely one of poorer young women.

Curiously, the teen birth rate was considerably higher in the United States in the early to mid-twentieth century than it is today. However, virtually every teen giving birth at that time was married. Rarely is that the case today, and fewer than a third of all biological fathers of a teen mother's baby are very involved with the baby and the mother.

In part because of this, babies of teenage mothers have a significantly greater chance of growing up in poverty than do babies of two-parent families or of single mothers older than twenty. Bearing a child as a teenager—and especially more than one child—confers similar economic disadvantages on the mother as well, for obvious reasons: because of child care needs, she is less likely to complete school or obtain higher paying jobs than are her older or married counterparts.

The national debate on how to address this concern swings between two extremes, with most Americans falling somewhere in the middle. On one side are those who preach absolute abstinence until marriage—the "just say no" approach. There is nothing wrong with encouraging abstinence; indeed, for most teenagers that is probably the wisest and safest course. However, it is wildly unrealistic to expect that preaching abstinence alone is going to solve the problems of sexually transmitted disease and pregnancy in teenagers.

On the other side is the argument that all teen sexual activity is natural and okay so long as the participants use safe sex practices, including effective contraception. In my view it is only logical that sexually active teens have easy access to sex education and contraceptive devices. However, it still makes sense to point out the benefits of abstinence, at least until the participants are older. Selling that concept to teens can be made easier by stressing the benefits of avoiding the emotional turmoil that can result when sexual activity occurs at too young an age. Baltimore has long had a problem with high rates of teen births. In fact, as recently as 1991, the city ranked first among major American cities, with approximately 12 percent of our teenage women under the age of nineteen giving birth each year.

One of the innovations the city health department chose to help address the problem was the provision of contraceptives in our school-based health centers. As noted earlier, Dr. Santelli initiated that program in 1986, putting Baltimore in the forefront nationally in contraceptive availability.

Six years later, when I started as health commissioner, I took it a step further in what proved to be the most controversial issue in my thirteen years in the position. It began innocently enough as a medical issue but soon pointed up my naiveté as a politician.

As a part-time physician at one of our school-based health centers I saw firsthand that unintended adolescent pregnancy was common. The most likely reason for a student to visit a school clinic was for a reproductive health issue. I quickly lost track of the number of times I saw fourteen-, fifteen-, and sixteen-year olds who became pregnant either because they didn't think they could get pregnant or because they forgot to take the pill every day.

Because I had a fair amount of experience with family planning issues, I was very aware of a long-acting contraceptive introduced in the United States in the late 1980s under the brand name Norplant. It is a system of five thin rods, each about one inch in length, which are implanted just under the skin of the inner surface of the upper arm. They slowly release a hormone that keeps the patient from ovulating—and thus from becoming pregnant—for about five years.

Norplant did have some fairly common side effects that would make it less desirable for some women, including headaches and weight gain. It also tended to reduce or eliminate periods, which some women found appealing but others found discomfiting—because they couldn't tell if they were pregnant or not. Also, of course, Norplant did not protect against HIV or other STDs, so a condom was still recommended.

At about the time that I started in my position as health commissioner—September 1992—Norplant was attracting considerable publicity in the press and women's magazines as a very desirable product, mainly because a woman didn't have to remember to take a pill every day. While spending time in our clinics, I was repeatedly asked by my female patients about the availability of this relatively new contraceptive. Since we were one of the very few cities in the country with school-based health centers that

IT IS WILDLY UNREALISTIC TO EXPECT THAT PREACHING ABSTINENCE ALONE IS GOING TO SOLVE THE PROBLEMS OF SEXUALLY TRANSMITTED DISEASE AND PREGNANCY IN TEENAGERS

provided family planning services, I decided to look into the option of providing Norplant to our teenagers, just as we did with the pill, diaphragms, and condoms.

After finding that the side effects were no more common among teens than adults and that Norplant was a most practical option for this notoriously noncompliant age group, I discussed with Mayor Schmoke the idea of introducing it in our high school centers. He was solidly behind it.

The first step was the formation of a group of experts to develop a plan on how to increase access to Norplant by teenagers across the city. One task for this group, composed mostly of local ob-gyns and teen health advocates, was to determine how each prescription of Norplant would be paid for. The up-front cost of a Norplant insertion was about $350 at the time—significantly higher than the $10 for a pack of contraceptive pills—although over the five year life of the implants, it would actually be less expensive than the pill.

The issue of access presented a major hurdle, as many teens in the city did not have insurance or Medicaid, both of which paid for Norplant insertions. (The Clinton administration's program to expand Medicaid coverage to significantly more youngsters—the Children's Health Insurance Program, or CHIP—was still years away.) But a local group, the Abell Foundation, agreed to help.

Ultimately, by viewing it as an issue of equity and choice, our group of experts agreed that the provision of Norplant to uninsured teens in school-based clinics and other community-based clinics such as Planned Parenthood was a sensible move.

In early December 1992, the Baltimore *Sun* published a front-page story profiling our Norplant program under the banner headline, "City Officials Planning to Promote Norplant." Within hours, I was caught up in a media maelstrom phenomenon for which I hadn't been prepared. Articles appeared in the *New York Times*, the *Washington Post*, and other major newspapers, followed quickly by a spate of editorials, almost all of which were very positive. Most noted that this was a bold approach to reducing Baltimore's teen birth rate, which at that time placed us among the top two cities in the country.

Thinking we were over the hump, we went back to the process of determining just how we would make Norplant available in the school health centers. Thanks to the Abell Foundation we had plenty of Norplant kits, so the next step was to come up with a protocol for how to do the insertions. We trained our clinicians not only in technical procedures but also in strongly emphasizing to the young women getting Norplant the need to use condoms to prevent STDs.

The final step was to inform the community—in this case the parents and staff of the six high schools with clinics. Meetings were set up with PTAs and staff in which our director of family planning and I presented information about Norplant and explained why we wanted to offer it in the schools. We were almost uniformly well received, so I reported back to the mayor that I thought it was quite reasonable to proceed.

Mayor Schmoke had one question before giving the final go ahead. Would parents of the individual patients be involved? Maryland, like most states, has a minor consent law, which prohibits requiring parents to be notified if their child is receiving family planning, mental health, or substance abuse services. However, in this situation, it wasn't so much the law we were concerned with as practical matters. For example, it would be hard for parents not to find out that their daughter had a Norplant insertion because of the bandage on her arm or, if the child was relatively thin, the visible rods beneath her skin.

We decided to make a real effort to encourage our prospective Norplant patients to talk to their parents and involve them in the decision. This proved very successful. With the first dozen patients, all had strong parental involvement, and several had their mothers attend the insertion process. The heavy dose of counseling on the need to use condoms was also very effective. A follow-up review of those first dozen young women showed that only one was diagnosed with an STD in the nine months after getting Norplant. This compared quite favorably with an expected rate of 35 percent based on our entire population of teens in our clinics. The review also determined that the vast majority of those patients reported using condoms when they had intercourse. Finally, and most importantly for these young women, not one got pregnant while on Norplant.

It was tempting then to echo Shakespeare's words "All's well that ends well." In fact, the end was still a long way off.

I performed the first Norplant insertion in mid-January of 1993, at the Paquin School—Baltimore's school for pregnant and parenting teens.

We chose this school for the initial dozen insertions for a couple of reasons: the principal was extremely supportive of the initiative and wanted everything possible for her students. And, being a school for girls who had already been pregnant, we thought it would be the least controversial site for the initial insertions.

As things went smoothly on the clinical side, they ran into rough seas on the political side. In late January, a small but vocal group of citizens began speaking out in opposition to our initiative. They claimed that we were targeting African American teenagers and excluding parents from the decision-making process. Neither of those claims was true, of course. However, in February, city councilman Carl Stokes introduced a resolution asking the city council to weigh in on whether Norplant should be made available in the school-based health centers.

Prior to that city council hearing all hell broke loose as our health issue exploded suddenly into a racial issue, with charges that I was trying to commit genocide. Threats were made against my life and the city's homicide squad surrounded our house for a week to provide protection. Some of the more populist preachers in the city had a field day with the whole thing, revving up their congregations to oppose Norplant. Seeing such controversy, the media didn't hesitate to jump on as well.

At the hearing, I sat through seven hours of testimony from dozens of citizens, many spewing hatred. Some claimed that I was trying to keep black children from being born, others that I didn't care if these girls got AIDS. Still more said we were coercing young girls into getting irreversible contraception that we would refuse to remove, while others, with pointed anti-Semitic references, said that I wouldn't do this to my own children.

All but one of those who testified in opposition to Norplant was male. As with abortion and other reproductive health issues, it's been my experience that men frequently arrogantly believe they know what is best when it comes to what's good for women.

The hearing was covered live by all of the local television stations and by a national network. The media onslaught continued after the hearing to the point that, by the end of the next month, I had done several dozen interviews with radio and television stations from all over the world, including England, Canada, Japan, and Germany.

In the meantime, Mayor Schmoke never wavered in his support.

"I supported Peter on that," he told Patrick McGuire. "He was absolutely right. But some ministers and many conservative political people didn't like it and thought he was using children as guinea pigs. Others were philosophically opposed to it.

"Peter needed support from me because it was an area where it would have been easy for him, as a white commissioner, to be demonized for experimenting on the black community. I met with the interdenominational ministerial alliance about it, some people from Baltimore United In Leadership Development, and parent groups. A lot of parent groups supported it. I had to encourage them to voice their support instead of being silent.

"That took a little bit of political activity. Peter was good at talking to the press and policy people in Washington about it. Folks from Washington were always looking over our shoulder on things like that because we received so much federal funding. We just couldn't afford to run afoul of them."

The mayor's behind-the-scenes work paid off. The furor died down within just a few weeks, and it became obvious to council members that, in spite of the negative remarks from the hearing, the general public in the city was in favor of our policy. A consensus was reached with the council, that Norplant wasn't to be promoted over other options and that we not use coercion—neither of which we had planned to do anyway. The council then voted down the resolution unanimously, with Councilman Stokes actually abstaining in the end.

We continued inserting Norplant in our school health centers for the next couple of years without any problems. The rate of side effects was lower than expected, as was the incidence of sexually transmitted infections. Not only did none of the girls get pregnant but most also decided to leave the implant in for the full five years. In fact, in subsequent years two of the young women who had gotten Norplant at the Paquin School came up to me on the street to thank me for providing it, as they were able to finish high school and get good jobs that they didn't think would have been possible if they had gotten pregnant again.

Norplant insertions fell off sharply throughout the country in the mid-1990s as the result of a class action suit filed over problems with removals in Chicago—a problem that we never had. However, we continue to provide long-term contraception in our school-based health centers by giving girls the option of Depo-Provera, an injection that prevents pregnancy for three months at a time. More than a thousand young women in our schools have availed themselves of this contraceptive. Although certainly not the only reason, I think it is clear that the provision of contraception in our school-based health centers helped Baltimore drop from having the highest teen birth rate in the country to the number 15 ranking: over the past twenty years, the city's teen birth rate dropped by more than 40 percent.

When I talk about this experience in lectures to public health graduate students today they often ask what I would have done differently with the Norplant issue. Honestly, I don't think any of the actions we took would be different. We did due diligence on the science of Norplant, we met with the right groups, we did the groundwork of discussing the proposal with parents and staff at the affected schools. And we listened to the most important group—the young women in these schools who had simply requested equal access to a contraceptive that those with insurance could get easily.

In retrospect, however, it was probably not the issue to cut my teeth on as the brand new, very young health commissioner. At the time, no one in the city really knew me, particularly in the African American community. Despite the fact that I obviously had gotten approval for our Norplant initiative from Mayor Schmoke, who is black, there was mistrust of my motives in the community. I firmly believe that had I proposed something similar ten years later, when I was more widely known for working to improve the health of all in the city, the initiative would have drawn little, if any, comment. The lesson: before proposing a potentially controversial initiative, understand that working to obtain the trust of the community is absolutely necessary.

IN 1997, ANOTHER NATIONAL TELEVISION PROGRAM had an impact on Baltimore and the city health department. Like *The Wire*'s exposure of the city's drug culture, the impact was a negative one for the city. But unlike *The Wire*, there seemed no urgent lessons to be learned, other than a painful reminder to the health commissioner that follow-up with subordinates is a most important principle of business management.

It was on *The Tonight Show* with Jay Leno that the lantern-jawed comedian let the world know that Baltimore had just earned the ignominious distinction of being the syphilis capital of the United States. In his monologue one night Leno showed a video of a highway sign proclaiming, "Welcome to Baltimore. Please fasten your condom."

Obviously it was not the kind of publicity a city is looking for in promoting tourism or economic development. Chagrined that we had achieved this notoriety, I immediately started working with our communicable disease staff to come up with a strategy to deal with the problem—and to deal with it quickly.

But how did the problem arise in the first place?

The epidemiology of syphilis, at least in Baltimore, is different from that of most of the more common STDs. Most of them, like gonorrhea and chlamydia, tend to affect younger individuals than does syphilis. In Baltimore, for example, the vast majority of gonorrhea and chlamydia cases occur in the thirteen-to-twenty-five age group, generally among teens and young adults who know their partner's name and address. That is key, as it makes it relatively easy for our disease trackers to both treat the patient and follow up with their partner or partners.

Syphilis is different. It tends to affect an older group—twenty-five- to forty-five-year-olds—and a much more difficult population to pin down. In our outbreak of syphilis, much of the transmission centered on a population predominantly involved with drugs. In fact, the disease was spreading as part of a trade of sex for drugs. Consequently, few of the affected patients knew who or where their partners were. Adding to the difficulty, at this time several of the city's most notorious high rise projects were torn down and the residents scattered throughout the city, resulting in new pockets of infection that needed to be addressed.

That made it much more difficult to break the cycle of transmission. When the reservoir of infected individuals in certain heavily affected parts of the city reaches a "tipping point," the outbreak begins spreading any- and everywhere. In just a couple of years, we went from our typical level of about 150 cases per year to a high of 662 cases in 1997 (or a rate of 101.3 cases per 100,000 population)—a full 5 percent of all cases reported in the United States that year.

Unfortunately, I wasn't fully aware of the increase until the Centers for Disease Control and Prevention (CDC) was about to announce our number 1 status. I was taken by surprise and was a bit on the defensive when reporters began asking how I could let this happen. I then remembered an assistant commissioner from our communicable disease staff pulling me aside several weeks back as I was hurrying from one meeting to another. He whispered that our syphilis numbers were getting high. Distracted, I asked him to put it in a memo and send it to me. But I got no memo, and the issue slipped my mind.

All very interesting, if you're an aficionado of best practices in management. Otherwise, the excuse did nothing to correct the syphilis outbreak. Chagrined, I took responsibility and began looking for a solution.

Our approach to reducing the syphilis rate was strategically targeted at the epidemiology of the outbreak and consisted of four parts. First, we increased the staff at our two STD clinics, where more than half of all patients with sexually transmitted diseases in the city are seen each year. In doing so, we hoped to avoid turning away any potential syphilis patients because of lack of capacity. In addition, because this was their area of expertise, our STD clinics were the best sites to properly identify and treat syphilis patients. Since syphilis is relatively rare, many providers haven't seen it before. We were getting cases where patients would come to our clinics with an obvious syphilitic lesion—a painless genital ulcer, called a chancre—that had been misdiagnosed a couple of weeks earlier in a community hospital emergency room as a fungal infection.

Second, we mounted an education campaign—of both providers and at-risk individuals, describing the increase in syphilis cases and what to look for as signs and symptoms. Third, realizing that the drug-related characteristics of many of our syphilis patients could result in their arrest, we established a "stat" lab for syphilis testing at the city's central booking facility, which processed one hundred thousand arrestees each year. This proved to have a great yield—about 25 percent of our new cases each year are now picked up through this lab.

Finally, recognizing that many of these syphilis patients neither had easy access to medical care nor would most of them be terribly likely to seek help, we knew we would simply have to resort to canvassing large chunks of the inner city. We trained our disease trackers in drawing blood and sent them to crack houses and other locations frequented by those most at risk for syphilis. There the trackers would draw blood and would bring in any person who tested positive for treatment.

This four-point initiative worked tremendously well. We achieved significant drops in our syphilis rates each year since 1997, dropping to only 115 cases in 2002 (an 84 percent drop from our peak of 662, for a rate of 19.3 cases per 100,000 population). It stood as the largest five-year drop of any American city since those numbers have been recorded. In practical terms, the "tipping point" phenomenon now played out in our favor. As the population of infected individuals became smaller and smaller, the likelihood of unsafe sexual practice leading to further transmissions became smaller as well. This lower rate of syphilis infection has continued to this day (in 2007, the most recent year with complete statistics, the rate was 20.9 cases per 100,000 population).

In retrospect, at a time when the role or even the need for government involvement in our lives is questioned by many of our political leaders, I view the measures we took regarding contraception and syphilis as a prime example of government's ability and responsibility to help citizens in need.

For years, the high rates of teen births and sexually transmitted diseases were often viewed by officials and citizens alike as intractable problems affecting the inner city. However, smart, targeted approaches to both issues resulted in dramatic reductions in each in a relatively short period of time, a tribute to a strategic public health policy implemented by dedicated professionals.

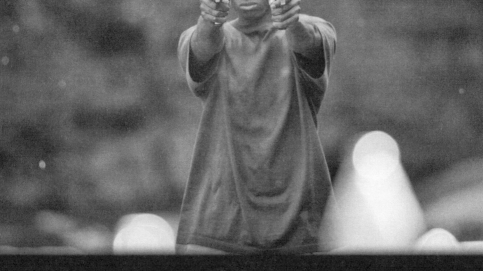

Cold-blooded drug lord Marlo Stanfield kills those who cross him and trains others to do the same. Citing a public health emergency enabled officials in Baltimore to prevent sales of ammunition to minors as a first step in reducing gun violence. THE WIRE/HBO ©

CHAPTER 9

FIREPOWER

SNOOP'S BERETTA, AVON'S HECKLER, AND OMAR'S MOSSBERG

As seen time after time on *The Wire,* an unwritten rule of power governs the world of drug dealers: guns solve problems. A simple pull of a trigger at point blank range and the problem instantly goes away. As Omar Little explains to Detective William "Bunk" Moreland, "The game is out there and it's either play or get played."

For the rest of us whose lives are degraded and endangered by the violent backsplash of a game of fools and sociopaths, the exact opposite of that unwritten rule has become our reality: problems are caused by guns.

On *The Wire,* whenever pride gets wounded, reason fails, or paranoia triumphs, guns are always at hand. For instance, when Bodie needs to prove himself to Stringer Bell, he aims a gun at his friend, Wallace. The latter's feeble cry of disbelief, "Yo, man, it's me," is no match for the bullet from Bodie's Taurus PT99.

That, by the way, is a model Omar is occasionally seen brandishing—though, clearly, his weapon of choice is the 12-gauge Mossberg 500 Cruiser. Which is not to say he isn't open-minded about other arms, for it's clear that Mr. Little sometimes would rather blast away with his Colt Gold Cup Match M1911A1. That's the same model handgun, of course, that Cheese wields in one of the final scenes of *The Wire*, just before Slim Charles bangs a bullet into his skull with a Sig Sauer P226. Not to be confused with the Sig Sauer P220, with which Chris shoots Prop Joe—incidentally the same type of gun used by O-Dog to kill Bodie. What goes around comes around and when it comes around to Omar, it's through the barrel of a Beretta 92FS wielded by twelve-year-old Kenard. That's the brand of hardware used on Snoop by Michael who then graduates to a Mossberg as an Omar copycat. Many other gun models make their appearance on *The Wire*, from your basic Glock 22 and 23 to Avon Barksdale's Heckler and Koch USP, to the somewhat exotic Makarov IJ70 carried by Bird. And, of course, there is Brother Mouzone's classic, James Bond-esque Walther PPK.380.

None of this detail comes from my own scant knowledge about the ways and means of firearms. I know very little about guns—although I do know quite a bit about their impact on people. So, when I recently came across a website describing in such reverent detail each and every deadly gun used on *The Wire*, I didn't know whether to laugh or to cry. To me, there's almost a farcical ring to the above litany of deadly arms, reminiscent somehow of the way boys on a corner in a more innocent time memorized and could instantly cite the specs on dozens of makes and models of automobiles or statistics about their favorite baseball or football star.

The wide-ranging armory on almost constant display in episodes of *The Wire* is but another carefully reported detail that gives the series its disturbing and coldly realistic air. Even viewers who can't tell an automatic from a revolver will come away certain that, whatever the weapons are, they are some very lethal guns.

They are guns, by the way, that most viewers would have no idea how to obtain, and yet they are always at hand even to twelve-year-old assassins. That's not a Hollywood contrivance. That's the way it is. I remember the day Mayor Schmoke declared a Take Back the Corner Day and asked various members of his cabinet to stand on a number of heavily used drug corners around the city to demonstrate our resolve. I spent my time on such a corner, within sight of the Johns Hopkins hospital, talking casually with kids who were dealing drugs, kids who felt no compunction about conducting business as usual in the midst of an effort specifically targeting them.

I asked one of the boys how hard it would be for me to get my hands on a gun. With great enthusiasm, this young teen began pointing out the houses up and down both sides of the intersecting streets where I could easily get a certain type of handgun for anywhere between thirty and a couple hundred dollars.

It continues to puzzle me that in the United States we seem to be willing to accept a level of violence between our citizens known only in countries experiencing a civil war. This violence occurs predominantly among two major groups: domestic violence between intimate partners and family members and violence between acquaintances, usually over criminal activity involving drugs.

An additional burden of violence occurs in crimes of passion between individuals, often teens and young adults who become involved in disputes over seemingly minor acts of "disrespect." There is more than enough of that kind of killing that takes place on the harsh streets of *The Wire.* Typical is the scene in Episode 38, Season 4, when Lex shoots Fruit, one of Marlo's lieutenants, because he was making time with Lex's girlfriend.

ON *THE WIRE,* WHENEVER PRIDE GETS WOUNDED, REASON FAILS, OR PARANOIA TRIUMPHS, GUNS ARE ALWAYS AT HAND

Speaking of Marlo, the cold-blooded sociopath was the hands-down master of the "disrespect equals a bullet in the head" attitude. In Episode 41 of Season 4, in a chilling foreshadowing of future violence, Marlo enters a corner market in west Baltimore. A security guard watches his every move. Marlo, very aware of the scrutiny, steals a handful of lollipops, slipping them into his pocket as he walks out of the store. The security guard confronts Marlo and says, "I know who you are . . . you act like you don't even know I'm there." To which Marlo casually responds, "I don't." Later in the episode there is a scene where Marlo's two hired assassins, Chris and Snoop, are in their truck, watching the corner store and the security guard. "What he do again?" asks Snoop. To which Chris answers, "Talked back."

By the end of the episode, the security guard is dead and his body hidden away in a nearby vacant house.

Unfortunately, acts of violence are more likely to result in death or severe injury in the United States than elsewhere because of the incredible prevalence of handguns. With more than 200 million guns in the hands of citizens, there are as many guns as there are adults.

In the United States, the debate over guns is rarely one of science or statistics but rather one of politics and propaganda. The "pro-gun" side, led by the powerful National Rifle Association, or NRA, uses the fear of victimization by predatory criminals to argue a need for easy access to guns among virtually all citizens.

The evidence supporting the NRA's propaganda is misleading. In fact, in spite of its strident advocacy of the self-defense rationale, individuals are many times more likely to use a gun to kill or injure themselves or a family member (through accident, suicide, or homicide) than to shoot an intruder. A perfect example is the well-known case of former New York Giants football star Plaxico Burress. He took a concealed handgun into a bar—presumably for self-defense—and then accidentally shot himself in the leg.

Unfortunately, the United States Supreme Court has made the challenge facing gun control advocates much harder in a pair of recent rulings. In 2008, the Supreme Court overruled the opinion of many constitutional legal scholars regarding the intent in the Second Amendment to grant citizens the right to bear arms. In *District of Columbia v. Heller*, the high court said the individual's right to bear arms was not limited by or connected to the right of a state to raise an armed militia. Two years later in its *McDonald v. Chicago* ruling, the court put restrictions on state and local governments' ability to limit the individual's right to bear arms.

In my view, those rulings dangerously distort the balance between an individual's right to protect one's self and property and the equally important, but now diminished, right of a community to reasonably decide how to weigh the rights of every citizen against its duty to protect those citizens.

But, rather than adding to the endless, no-win arguments between those who support gun control and those who don't, it would be far more productive to push for gun control as a public health measure.

There is a precedent for this approach in the campaign against smoking. Fighting over the right of individuals to smoke produced little movement. Legislation and lawsuits controlling access to cigarettes were successful only when tobacco use was portrayed by anti-tobacco advocates as a major public health problem. This claim was easily supported by the data—including the statistic that tobacco use is the largest single cause of preventable death, responsible for more than 450,000 deaths in this country each year.

A similar approach can be taken with firearms, by portraying gun violence as the public health epidemic it is and using statistics to back up this claim. This, too, should be easy to do: for example, homicides and suicides by gun kill more Americans between the ages of fifteen and twenty-four than any cause other than accidents.

Gun control advocates also need to concretely rebut one of the NRA's most misleading slogans: "Guns don't kill people; people kill people." What utter foolishness. It is certainly no secret that person-to-person violence has been taking place since Cain killed Abel. But can anyone seriously doubt that if violence between individuals was still limited to blunt objects or knives, fewer arguments would end in death? Or that tighter controls on access to guns would result in fewer people killing people—whether with malice or by accident?

As for the legitimacy of owning a handgun for the purposes of self-defense, the fear people may have for their safety is understandable. Fear is a constant in our society, and people's vulnerability to it is exploited in numerous ways from movies to TV to political gamesmanship. If some "grandma" were to use her Glock semiautomatic handgun to scare off an intruder, the NRA would make sure we never heard the end of it. In real life, it very rarely happens. When fearful people buy guns, the fear doesn't magically go away. The real fear is that fearful people may injure themselves or loved ones with a handgun they often don't know how to use or handle in calm—let alone stressful—situations. Such fears are the legitimate basis for society paying taxes to field a professional and well-trained police force.

I know there are many responsible gun owners who take the ownership of a weapon seriously enough to be trained in safe handling practices and who take every precaution to keep it out of reach of children. But let's be honest. Those gun owners are not the majority of private citizens who buy handguns for their safety. And, reflecting back to the ludicrous litany of firepower found at the beginning of this chapter, owning a handgun for defense is one thing, but what legitimate purpose is served by owning a submachine gun, an assault rifle, or any exotic, beyond-the-basics handgun?

Yet, gun advocates will cite chapter and verse on the need for overwhelming firepower and tell horrific stories of the poor grandma, armed only with a six-shot revolver who was attacked by a squad of street thugs armed with automatic assault rifles. Thus, goes the argument, granny should have the right to buy a submachine gun for her self-defense. If we really need machine guns to protect ourselves, our society is far worse off than I or anyone is aware of. The truth is we likely would be happier and healthier in dealing with irrational fears by confronting them and trying to better understand ourselves than by the self-delusion of needing a gun to keep us safe in a moment of life-threatening danger.

WITH MORE THAN 200 MILLION GUNS IN THE HANDS OF CITIZENS, THERE ARE AS MANY GUNS AS THERE ARE ADULTS

To that end, I believe we should make the sale of such guns and ammunition in urban areas as difficult as possible. Pushing that envelope may be politically unfeasible on a national level. Although the recent Supreme Court decisions make it harder, efforts to more stringently regulate access to guns and ammunition can be successful at the local level, and in Baltimore we are moving in that direction.

FOR DECADES BALTIMORE HAS ENDURED one of the highest murder rates of any city in the nation, including a stretch from the mid-1980s to 2000 with more than three hundred murders a year. In the 2000s, homicide (not accidents, as for the rest of the nation) was the leading cause of death for fifteen- to twenty-four-year-olds. In 2010, even with a reduction in its number of homicides to 223, the city still ranked fifth in murders in the country, with more than half of those homicide victims under thirty.

As one would expect, the preponderance of these homicides are committed with guns. And analyses of fatal and nonfatal shootings show that the vast majority of victims of gunshots in the city are involved in some way with the drug trade. It is striking, however, to find little sense of urgency or outrage in the city over these numbers. Was it because these victims are overwhelmingly young, male, and black? Is it because many people are in a state of voluntary denial—it's not happening to them and their kin but only to "gang bangers"? Or maybe it is simply a matter of resignation because of the city's long history of high homicide rates. The only real response, at least publicly, has been the occasional "stop the killing" march at the site of a homicide, usually organized by a local preacher.

In 2002, in an effort to seize the initiative, I went back to the Johns Hopkins Bloomberg School of Public Health where I had done my residency in preventive medicine. I met with one of my mentors from those days, Steve Teret, and a colleague, Nancy Lewin. Teret, an attorney and public health policy expert, heads the Johns Hopkins Center for Gun Policy and Research. Both Nancy and Steve offered several suggestions to get at the gun issue, some highly innovative, some radical, and some quite practical. The most promising involved using the legal powers of the commissioner of health to intervene in threats to the public health as a tool to get at the gun issue.

Baltimore's city charter grants very broad authority to the health commissioner to both define a public health threat and to chart a course of action to deal with it. Usually this authority is used by a health commissioner to bring food handlers into compliance, as in the case of the Super Pride chain of supermarkets described in chapter 2 or to take charge of an issue involving communicable diseases, as in the school immunization effort in chapter 7. In each of those situations, I deemed the issue at hand serious enough to qualify as a public health emergency. When we decided to tackle gun violence, the city government was saying that this type of violence, especially among youth, was so widespread that it equaled a public health emergency. It was an unusual and controversial step, as fewer than one in five health commissioners nationwide have used their powers to intervene in gun violence.

Our specific response to the epidemic of youth gun violence was also unusual. If we could have legally targeted the sale of handguns, we would have. However, while Maryland law prohibits possession or sale of handguns and ammunition to anyone under twenty-one, there is also a state preemption law that places limits on what local jurisdictions can do in terms of gun control. Essentially, they can't do very much.

Undeterred, we decided to focus instead on handgun ammunition sales to minors—on the rather obvious theory that without bullets a gun can't shoot anyone. At first glance, it appeared that the state preemption law forbade us from going in this direction. But in discussions with the Baltimore Police Department and with police commissioner Ed Norris, we learned that ammunition sales to minors were ongoing at many local hardware stores and other outlets and were an issue of great concern to the police. Yet sellers of this ammunition to minors were rarely arrested or prosecuted. Why? More quirks in the law. While prohibited under state and federal law, ammunition sales to minors were, for some reason, not subject to the same licensing requirements as gun sales. There were also no specific zoning laws in Baltimore governing ammunition sales in certain areas; therefore little enforcement was going on.

Meanwhile, in his legal research, Steve Teret found a potential opening in the preemption law. While it prohibited local jurisdictions from involvement with gun control, it also listed a small number of exceptions. One of them stated that a local firearm initiative aimed at minors would be legal.

Thus, using the authority of my office—and in conjunction with the Baltimore Police Department and the Johns Hopkins University—I declared the illegal sale of ammunition to minors in the city a public health threat, and we launched our Youth Ammunition Initiative.

The first step was to identify the targets of our initiative—made possible by information supplied by the police department. Then, with the support of the police special operations squad we planned a series of "stings," recruiting police cadets under the age of twenty-one to make purchases of ammunition at several stores.

In the urban core of Baltimore, one of the few places ammunition is sold is at corner hardware stores, so that is where we targeted our stings. But there were complications almost immediately. Many types of ammunition can be used interchangeably in weapons whose use is both prohibited by minors (like semiautomatic pistols) and not prohibited (like certain hunting rifles). Thus, our cadet buyer couldn't just enter a hardware store and ask for a certain type of ammunition.

One solution was for the cadet to show a prohibited weapon to the store clerk while asking for the ammunition. This was quickly abandoned out of concern it would be too risky for the cadet. The clerk or store owner might suspect a holdup that could result in an owner shooting the cadet in "self-defense." Having the cadet state what type of weapon he needed the bullets for wouldn't work either, because there wouldn't be adequate evidence for a successful case. We finally came up with the idea that the teen would bring a picture of a prohibited weapon while asking for the ammunition—we felt this was evidence that would hold up in court.

In June and July 2002, stings were attempted at a handful of hardware stores in the city, chosen for their proximity to recent homicides. Buys were actually made by our cadet at one of them. After three successful buys on different days at this hardware store in west Baltimore, a joint police and health department search and seizure raid was conducted. I followed the special operations police team clad in bulletproof vests into the store with a senior staffer, Melisa Lindamood, who had helped coordinate the project. The team served its search warrant on the store owner and cited the clerk who had illegally sold the ammunition to the cadet.

The police seized dozens of boxes of ammunition, including armor-piercing bullets and even one box that advertised the possibility of buying individual bullets. It is this real-life scenario that runs so counter to NRA propaganda about responsible gun and ammunition sales.

While the police completed their search, I met with the owner of the family-run hardware shop to present him with a health commissioner's order closing his store for being a threat to the public's health by endangering minors. This was apparently the first time in the country that a store was closed for selling ammunition illegally by health department fiat, and it gained national attention.

In anticipation of these raids, we had written a set of regulations that would govern our handling of stores found to sell to minors. Conforming to the exception from the state's preemption law, our regulations explained why we were closing the store and laid out requirements the store would need to meet to protect minors before it could reopen.

Our approach from the start was to stop these ammunition sales to minors, not simply to cite merchants who were involved. Our motivation was much more on the side of prevention than punishment. At the outset, the owners were allowed to appeal the closure of their hardware store, which they did immediately, and a hearing was held the following day at the health department.

At the hearing, which I conducted, the special operations officers from the police department testified to the facts. The owners were allowed to comment and brought a lawyer who was very pleasant (he was actually the owner's relative and didn't normally handle these types of cases). He didn't bother cross-examining the officers, who presented an ironclad case. I concluded that the evidence was clear that the store had violated the department of health regulations we had earlier promulgated and, consequently, the closure was upheld.

The store owners conceded their guilt, and, by regulation, were then offered two options that would allow them to reopen: (1) they could cease selling all ammunition, period or (2) they could sell ammunition but would be required to keep a log with copies of photo IDs with all receipts for these sales to insure that they were checking for proof of legal age.

During the hearing, the store owners had made a point of how they were a long-standing family-owned business, devoted to the community. I appealed to them to take the first option. If they truly cared about the community they served—one beset by very high rates of violent crime— they would stop contributing to the problem by ceasing ammunition sales, especially since they were one of the few stores selling such products for miles around. I was disappointed when their sense of responsibility to the community took a back seat to the desire to continue to make a profit from selling ammunition: they took the second option.

The combined police, academic research, and health operation received a significant amount of local media coverage during which we stated that such innovative actions would continue. Our hope was that the sting— small and relatively symbolic as it was—might make other careless or unscrupulous business owners think twice before doing business as usual.

A postscript to the story: I went back to the store a few months after they reopened to make sure they were keeping the appropriate log with photo IDs. I was pleasantly surprised to find that rather than dealing with that hassle and the likely recurring inconvenience of police or health department visits, the owners decided to follow our first option and stop selling all ammunition, period. In the end, we actually did achieve our objective.

ENCOURAGED BY THE SUCCESS of our first regulatory foray into publicly defining violence as a public health issue, the health department generated three important pieces of legislation—with the backing of the mayor and police commissioner. By the way, that cumbersome state law preempting any local law limiting sales of guns or ammunition was not an accident. Over a period of years, the NRA made a concerted effort to get states to pass such laws. With them in place, the NRA had only to fight battles in fifty state capitals, rather than in hundreds or even thousands of city halls. Thus, one of our legislative proposals—at the state level—was to remove the local preemption from Maryland's gun and ammunition laws. It was unlikely to pass on the first try because of heavy lobbying by the NRA and its allies, but we felt it worth pursuing.

Unfortunately, this effort stalled, but we were successful at the local level, with two city council bills. One mandated that all sellers of ammunition make and retain copies of photo IDs for all ammunition sales, the same requirement we applied to the "stung" store. This met the exception to state law since it was done to protect minors from obtaining illegal ammunition. Just as important, it serves as a useful tool for police, giving them reasonable cause to obtain a search warrant in tracing felons or those with open warrants who have illegally attempted to buy ammunition.

In addition, we introduced a city ordinance to limit gun and ammunition sales within set distances from parks, churches, schools, and public gathering places. Enactment of or changes to zoning law is a powerful strategy for localities in bypassing preemptive state laws. Courts have tended to uphold local decisions about where certain activities can be sited.

The city council unanimously passed both bills, and the mayor used the signing ceremony as an opportunity to highlight our innovative approach to defining gun violence as a public health issue.

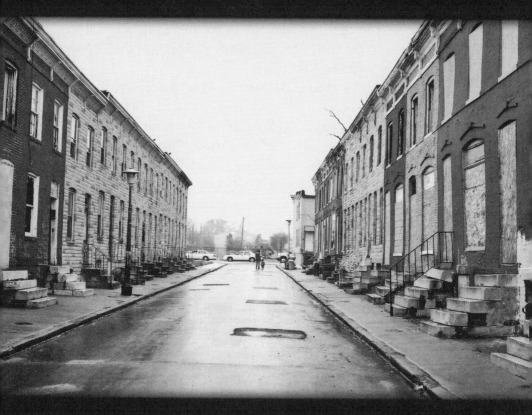

Place matters. Children growing up in poverty on streets such as this one on *The Wire* and experiencing the neglect and violence portrayed in the series have a dramatically harder time succeeding in school and in life than do those with more stable surroundings. THE WIRE/HBO ©

CHAPTER 10

PLACE MATTERS

WHY DIDN'T BODIE JUST LEAVE?

NEAR THE END OF *THE WIRE*'S SECOND SEASON we catch up with Preston "Bodie" Broadus, a teenage crew chief of young hoppers on a west Baltimore drug corner. A fierce, though at times uncertain, boy, Bodie is a streetwise escapee from a common form of dysfunctional family in a drug- and poverty-ridden neighborhood: absent, unknown father; absent, most likely drugged-out mother; unseen and likely overwhelmed grandmother.

Bodie would be just another bad guy in a standard police drama, but he is painted here in multiple shades of gray. He tries very hard to maintain the only identity he has been able to carve out of street chaos, that of loyal soldier in the drug wars. But when his leader, Avon Barksdale, goes off to prison, souls like Bodie are left adrift, their anchor of loyalty dislodged, their sense of self-worth and identity in doubt.

Across several previous episodes we have seen in Bodie's gruff exterior and tough-guy spitting prowess a poignant but inevitable deterioration from rough innocence to acts of violence. Yet, in Bodie's case, it is not the cold-blooded violence of a Marlo Stanfield. Bodie's appeal as a somewhat good bad guy comes from our feeling that he is unsettled by killing his friend Wallace—a hit ordered by the cold-blooded Stringer Bell and carried out by an eager-to-prove-himself loyalist.

We sense that Bodie has a conscience and a street level feel for what is really right and what is not. So he marches on, feeling that his life holds no other option. He is one of the many gunslingers on these cheerless streets who believe they will be dead before the age of thirty.

In Episode 22, Season 2, a gang of independent drug dealers launches an attack on Bodie's drug corner. Guns are produced on both sides and, contrary to the precise choreography of a Hollywood shootout or the faux realism of a video game, this one plays out almost as farce. Errant shots from badly aimed automatics fly in every direction, a perfect display of the kind of fantasy gunfight eight-year-old boys might stage with toy guns and heavy drama.

But these are real guns with real bullets. And while most of them hit no one, a stray round goes through the wall of an adjacent house and kills a nine-year-old boy being readied for school by his mother. That dead nine-year-old and the living Bodie share a common curse that has been cast on them by a kind of social predestination. What *The Wire* shows, intentionally or not, is that given the cruel fact of where they were born and where they live, the tragedy of their ruined lives is an almost predictable outcome.

If I learned one truth in my years as health commissioner in Baltimore, one of the poorest communities in the country, and now in nearby Howard County, one of the wealthiest, it is this: almost to the exclusion of everything else, place matters. If you live in an area with a solid education system, jobs that pay a living wage, access to health care, and decent housing, you, as an individual, are going to have a healthier, higher social status. All of which translates into well-being for you and the citizens of your community.

Growing up safe and healthy, and being able to go to school and actually learn, is often determined not by race or genes or a can-do attitude but by social and environmental factors. Look at inner city Baltimore, for example. There you will find a huge population of overweight children, a dismaying lack of recreational facilities, entire sections of the city without supermarkets (making them, essentially, food deserts), schools where children can't and don't learn, a lack of jobs and their pathway to making an honest living, and neighborhood streets that often become a drug-infested war zone. These problems are all related and reflect the social determinants for the future lives of the children and adults who live there.

More proof that the socioeconomic status of a neighborhood affects the lives of those who live there can be found in the results of the Program for International Student Assessment (PISA). It tests the reading, math, and science skills of fifteen-year-olds in the most developed countries of the world. If you listen to the media, you might be under the impression that the performance of American students falls well below the level of students in most developed countries. While that is technically correct, you will see a very different picture if you separate American school performance by the socioeconomic status of a student's family. Consider that, on the one hand, in American public schools where more than 75 percent of the students live in households below the federal poverty level, academic performance is worse than in all but one country, Finland, on the PISA test. On the other hand, students from American schools where less than 10 percent of students come from households below the poverty level, have performance rates better than students in any other country. Place matters.

IF I LEARNED ONE TRUTH IN MY YEARS AS HEALTH COMMISSIONER IN BALTIMORE AND NOW IN NEARBY HOWARD COUNTY, IT IS THIS: PLACE MATTERS

We can do every assessment of health that there is—we can find out that people are obese or they don't have access to medical care or they live in unsafe housing. But the typical liberal social programs that aim to prevent these problems are actually secondary prevention. Trying to reduce the consequences of the environment in which kids have been brought up without changing the negative aspects of that environment—without improving the social determinants—is almost hopeless.

One approach to addressing the pervasive poverty of place is to bring economic development directly to these neighborhoods. This can be done in a variety of ways:

- Offer tax breaks to businesses that locate in these communities and hire local residents.

- Offer low interest loans to encourage start-up businesses by community residents.

- Provide training to ensure that career ladders are available. For example, construction companies that relocate to an economically distressed area could provide training in lead paint abatement for entry level workers. They would therefore become a certified lead paint abatement specialist, a credential that will command significantly higher wages.

- Encourage recovery programs to tap into the skills of their patients or residents—even to provide training—so they themselves can run the various businesses of the organization, all of which are designed to help troubled citizens get back on their feet. (A very successful such program is run by the Delancey Street organization in San Francisco.)

Too often, however, politicians attempt a "trickle down" approach, favoring downtown-based economic efforts over neighborhood-based approaches. Not only have these top-down efforts failed to improve the economic situations of the have-nots, they also breed resentment and distrust of the political leaders by those in the poorer neighborhoods.

A glaring example of this tendency to advance the desires of the corporate interests to the neglect of needy neighborhoods came with the staging of a Grand Prix race in downtown Baltimore. Run Labor Day weekend of 2011, this three-day event received millions of dollars in public subsidies, even though the event sponsors admitted the race would not make money. Why would the city waste exorbitant amounts of precious resources to put on an event of both questionable economic or long-term value to the city? Why not channel these resources into job development activities to directly benefit members of vulnerable communities—permanent living-wage jobs, not the short-term low-paying hourly jobs that the tourism industry "creates"? Simply put, it seems clear that the economic powers-that-be aren't interested in the city's neighborhoods or long-term economic growth and that they attach far more value to the prestige that attracting the Grand Prix brings to themselves and the city.

Another promising approach to changing dysfunctional environments is to literally move some residents out of these neighborhoods and into communities with better opportunities (schools, jobs, housing, health). One such effort, a federal program called Moving to Opportunity (MTO), was implemented in Baltimore, Boston, New York, Chicago, and Los Angeles. However, the program ended unceremoniously in Baltimore, due to strident "not in my neighborhood," or NIMBY, concerns that carried definite racial overtones. Still, a partial settlement of the American Civil Liberty Union's suit over the abrupt cessation of MTO provided some relief. It required the United States Department of Housing and Urban Development to fund—and the city to provide—special vouchers to 2,100 families in impoverished areas (residents of inner-city high rises slated for demolition) to move to suburban, middle-class neighborhoods, predominantly in counties surrounding the city of Baltimore. Evidence accumulated over the ensuing decade in MTO's five pilot cities was generally positive.

Several comprehensive studies show that families did better in their new communities with respect to self-sufficiency, educational achievement, feelings of safety, child and parent health, and health inequities.

Unfortunately, these innovative approaches are attempted far too infrequently. Instead, we seem always to be chasing the tail of the problem. We will close city swimming pools in the middle of summer heat waves because of budget shortages, yet maintain excessively high levels of policing in poor neighborhoods, where having a place for children to swim not only keeps an idle mind busy but gets rid of pent-up energy. Why not deal with the main social determinants of health and socioeconomic well-being, which, in turn, will decrease the number of problematic people perpetrating antisocial behavior that requires more police?

Instead we see the all-too-common priority of hiring more police to chase criminals who are being churned out regularly in our most depressed communities, people who never should have become criminals in the first place. Shortly after becoming health commissioner in Baltimore, I became very involved with an initiative that attempted to break this endless cycle of chasing our tails by improving child health and wellness in poor city neighborhoods. The funder—the Robert Wood Johnson Foundation—solicited participation from private community groups in several large cities including Baltimore in 1992. They said, essentially, "We know your city has problems and we all know what kids need to grow up safe and healthy. So why isn't it happening?"

It set in motion a most unusual campaign that has attacked the problem from a radically different angle than anything tried previously in Baltimore. The campaign, under the leadership of experienced community organizer Hathaway Ferebee, is called Safe and Sound. I've frequently invited Ferebee to speak to my public health students.

"The real problem in too many cities," Ferebee says, "is the lack of opportunity for people to be successful. When you have opportunity, life turns out better, period. So many folks in Baltimore City just do not have the basic opportunity. They grow up in conditions that a human being can't really grow in. By design, behaviors that are unhealthy will manifest themselves in these environments."

That idea of "design" is central to the Safe and Sound philosophy. It argues that the way that we have allowed city neighborhoods to deteriorate into places of poverty and crime has been reactive instead of proactive. The Safe and Sound approach is to agree up front on a fundamental issue. If we, as a community, could change the way we devote resources to address problems in the city, then people could grow up safe, healthy, and educated and move into adulthood ready to take responsibility and live a normal life.

Ferebee talks about the "cradle to prison pipeline" theory. This theory suggests that where you are born and raised determines whether you will have the opportunities you need to live a healthy, productive life or whether you will land in prison. So, Safe and Sound looks at the environment, not the person. It argues that public policy in our cities anticipates or expects that certain groups of people in Baltimore City—primarily people of color—will inevitably end up in trouble.

"It's so easy to get in trouble in this city," says Ferebee. "The opportunities for staying out of trouble are so damn low. It's often crazy in the streets. Imagine living there and then being a good citizen. Think of the kind of behavior you must deploy in those neighborhoods. In a lot of ways the kind of actions people take are very rational. They're for survival but they also land them in jail."

The conditions of an environment, she adds, can shape a person's life expectations and even the ways one might respond to such conditions. "In any environment the way of acting and thinking becomes the norm," she says. "Thus, from the point of view of those lucky enough to live in an environment of opportunity, the choices made by people in an environment of poverty and low opportunity will often look stupid and lazy."

In other words, why didn't Bodie just get his act together and escape, maybe become a doctor or a teacher? Ferebee likes to confront this issue with the metaphor of a garden.

"Let's say you had a garden and ten seeds," she says. "Four of the seeds get no water, but six do. The six bloom and look pretty. You look at the four and say something is wrong with those seeds. So you give them a little bit of water, a little bit of plant food. Maybe a stick comes up. You say 'Why did I waste my money on those four? Why did I put that extra plant food in there?' When they start to die you think, well, I could put them in a hot house, but that costs even more money. And so you start to get irritated and you say 'Why couldn't you do as well as these other seeds?'"

The Wire seems perfectly attuned to this idea that people adapt and respond to their own environment with highly predictable results. In real life, because the results in areas of poverty and crime are so predictable our state and city budgets end up responding to the predictability of failure.

Safe and Sound rails against this "business as usual" approach, where public policy perpetuates what *The Wire* represented. Rather than blaming people for living in some of the most horrific situations imaginable and acting as if their way of behavior is the norm, Safe and Sound envisions changing the way we operate—and the way we allocate our public funds—by supporting healthy development as the norm and predicting success instead of failure.

But failure, says Ferebee, gets our attention and has led to policies built around expecting more failure. Consequently, the city spends a disproportionate and unreasonable amount on crime control. "Essentially," she says, "they are saying we know you're going to commit a crime. We're ready for you."

We need to stop spending money on unnecessary Grand Prix races and instead spend the money on opportunities and improving the environments in which children are raised.

AMONG THE "BUSINESS AS USUAL" PRACTICES Ferebee decries, is the almost unchallenged theory that crime control creates safe communities. But while public safety is fundamental to a community, she says, "you really don't get that through crime control, but through basic opportunities."

WHERE YOU ARE BORN AND RAISED DETERMINES WHETHER YOU WILL HAVE THE OPPORTUNITIES YOU NEED TO LIVE A HEALTHY, PRODUCTIVE LIFE OR WHETHER YOU WILL LAND IN PRISON

When a juvenile does something wrong, the norm is to put that child in penal custody instead of finding an opportunity for a more constructive intervention. The state spends $43 million a year to confine an average of five hundred juveniles convicted of nonviolent crimes. That's an average of $86,000 a year per young person. Once released, three out of four of those juveniles become repeat offenders.

Looking at the way the state conducted its business, Safe and Sound raised money to create interventions that would produce a better outcome than incarceration. It made a deal with the state that if their outcomes were better, the state would continue to pay for it and share the savings.

That successful intervention, begun in 2005, is called the Maryland Opportunity Compact (MOC) and is still operating. It took forty of the five hundred juveniles incarcerated each year and, rather than confine them, provided them with intensive multisystemic family therapy. That includes counseling for the family and all of its children, as well as helping parents deal with parenting issues and their child's behavior problems. It also provides the juvenile offender with a paid apprenticeship program, education, and continuous employment.

The cost of MOC is $20,000 a year per juvenile. It has saved the state $14 million so far. To date its success rate is 92 percent, with fewer than one in ten participants becoming a repeat offender.

The success of that program and other Safe and Sound initiatives had much to do with understanding that input from people other than professional organizers and social policy experts was critical.

"Just as we wanted city government to stop doing business as usual," says Ferebee, "we wanted people in affected neighborhoods to start thinking differently. We knew that if we started by asking people 'what are your problems?' we'd likely get a list of problems. The standard approach would then be to perhaps suggest a remedial program here and a drug treatment program there and so on. But we weren't after the standard. We decided that if we said to people 'what would you like?' we'd still be getting down to specifics but from a new angle that could be linked to an objective and a strategy."

Over a period of about a year the campaign engaged with hundreds of stakeholders and ordinary citizens who wanted to help. Safe and Sound launched an intensive neighborhood campaign, recruiting three hundred young people ages fifteen to eighteen to serve as our corps of youth ambassadors. The program trained them on how to use a megaphone and armed them with a list of suggested strategies for converting hopes into reality. Their job was to stand on street corners and go door to door generating discussions with neighbors around the various strategies. All of this as a way of promoting attendance at Baltimore's Promise, a large-scale forum we had planned for the city's arena.

The students and their teammates were immediately enthusiastic. They would stand on corners playing African drums and encouraging people to come over and say, "What are you doing?"

When the day of the convention rolled around organizers were stunned when seven thousand people showed up. It was extraordinary, essentially a seven thousand member focus group. Once inside the arena everyone was given a ballot and after some discussion they voted for the most important priorities by ranking them. That vote established the priorities for the Safe and Sound campaign.

The campaign then established ten goals based on the results of that vote. It sent teams of people to various cities to look at different kinds of programs that were achieving results in one or more goal areas. On each team was a young person, a community activist, a business person, a government representative, and a foundation official. They were required to eat two meals together on their trip. The first one came before seeing whoever they were going to visit and the second one was after the visit. They then had to come back to us and tell the campaign whether they would recommend that we look into that program some more. If they did, then Safe and Sound would take it from there to further investigate.

ONE OF THOSE TEAMS STRONGLY RECOMMENDED a program they'd visited in Boston called Ceasefire. Started in 1996 by David Kennedy, then of the John F. Kennedy School of Government at Harvard, Ceasefire worked very closely with the Boston Police Department to successfully target and bring to justice the most dangerous and violent of the city's criminals.

The Ceasefire premise held that in most high crime urban areas, criminal behavior, ranging from drug dealing to murder, originates among a small core of offenders. The idea is to target and prosecute the most violent of that core group of criminals and to use their fate as an object lesson as to what would soon happen to other troublemakers in town if they didn't get out of the crime business.

It almost sounds too simple to be practical, yet this plan worked, not only in Boston but in Baltimore as well.

To that end, Hathaway Ferebee's task was to build trust and support at the community level, while the office of the Baltimore state's attorney assigned a tough, energized assistant prosecutor named Kim Morton to the tricky task of unifying the law enforcement element.

"The first thing we all did," says Morton, "was agree to meet together every week. We brought all of our forces to bear—outstanding warrants, pending cases, anything we had on any of these people. We started to remove the anonymity from the action. At the end of the day, we found we were all dealing with the same folks."

After police had arrested a couple of ringleaders, Morton's office began phoning anyone in that geographical area suspected of some kind of violent crime or being engaged in narcotic activity. Those people were ordered to attend a group meeting with Ferebee and Morton where something in the nature of a riot act was read.

"We let them know that we knew what was going on," she said. "Most of them had other things pending in the legal system. We told them that for the first time in their lives when they walk into the courthouse, we will know who they are. And I might have thirty cases on my docket, and I can't try them all but I can make it a personal point that every time I get something with you involved, it goes to trial the first time in."

Morton and Ferebee would then tell them that this meeting was a warning. "If they so much as stubbed a toe illegally," she said, "not only would they be caught, so would everybody in their crew.

"We told them 'If you are the most violent community in Baltimore, then you will get the attention of all the law enforcement agencies. We promise. We will come in and get every last one of you *and* your buddies. We will confiscate all of the stuff you bought with ill-gotten gains.'"

Usually local ministers and some of the offender's neighbors attended these meetings and confronted the offenders, saying that this is the way it was going to be. Because the plan had total buy-in from the U.S. and state's attorneys, they knew this wasn't an idle threat. And while Morton used the promise of prosecution as a stick, she also brought out the carrot. That was me. I was introduced and told them that we were also there to help. I told them if anyone wanted to enter drug treatment I would get them into a program within twenty-four hours. Several offenders in each group took advantage of the offer.

Even so, after one of the first of these warning sessions, more than half of those invitees were arrested for another offense. As promised they were prosecuted to the full extent allowed. By the time a second group heard the warning, the number of those arrested was cut down considerably.

Over a nine month period Morton's office conducted five operations that brought down 147 offenders. In the two neighborhoods targeted in these initial stages of the initiative residents marveled at the quiet that had settled over the streets. A woman in Park Heights said, "It's like something happened."

Morton said the experience not only galvanized community and police commitment to the logic of doing business a new way, it changed her mind as well.

"I began to feel that there are very few criminals born. Some people I figure are just born insane and they're just going to do what they want. For the most part, a criminal is created and you have to approach that problem from both ends. Until I got involved in this work, I honestly didn't look at it like that. I thought, 'If you broke the law, you should go to jail.' But there's more to it than that."

And speaking of an approach from the other end, Morton related a story about a raid conducted by police at a house in Baltimore. When she stepped into the living room, she found several young children playing.

"There was a dead cat on the floor," she said. "And it had been there a while and was starting to decompose. And these kids are walking around it. In their living room. I mean, when you are raised and that is your reality . . . I just couldn't believe they lived this way. There were six little kids living in that house. You begin to appreciate that arresting your way out of this is never ever going to happen."

THE TRIAL RUN OF BALTIMORE'S VERSION of Ceasefire in two troubled neighborhoods—Park Heights and Cherry Hill—proved successful, even to the point where the Greater Baltimore Committee (equivalent to a big money, corporate chamber of commerce) put money into its continued growth. Despite this, when Kurt Schmoke left office as mayor in 1999, the future for the initiative was not bright. The Safe and Sound approach contradicted the political agenda of the new mayor, Martin O'Malley. He had campaigned on a tough, anticrime platform of zero tolerance. Clearly, he wanted to solve the problem through arrests even though the previous police chief—a supporter of the initiative—had said it was impossible to solve the drug problem with that kind of approach.

Under O'Malley's administration, police sweeps with large numbers of arrests became the norm in the city. In fact, the Maryland General Assembly a few years later passed a law expunging the records of thousands of people who had been arrested in those sweeps but later were released without being charged. Many complained they had been innocent bystanders caught in the right place at the wrong time. In 2006 alone, twenty-one thousand people were arrested but not charged.

Ultimately, Baltimore's version of Ceasefire never grew to the point where its track record was long enough that its unqualified success could be argued. Eventually it died for lack of support, a program that never got beyond its nascent stage because of a political agenda. It was an unfortunate ending for a program that focused like a laser on the most violent criminals in the most violent places in Baltimore, rather than simply casting a wide net to scoop up hordes of nonviolent offenders. The resulting savings in police costs could then have been used to improve the conditions of the neighborhoods—changing places for the better—ensuring that fewer violent criminals would come from them in the future.

Two kinds of lead are responsible
for the death of everyone's favorite
bad guy Omar Little: the bullet from
a handgun and paint dust from the
house of his twelve-year-old killer,
Kenard. Lead poisoning can result
in irreversible brain damage, which
can predispose a person to violent
behavior. THE WIRE/HBO ©

CHAPTER 11

OF PAINT AND GUNS

DID OMAR DIE OF LEAD POISONING?

WHAT IS THERE ABOUT OMAR LITTLE, the menacing, street-hardened murderer from *The Wire,* that makes him such a paradoxically appealing character? How is it that among all the violent gun-blazing dealers and schemers plying the drug trade on the streets of west Baltimore, viewers of *The Wire* tend to view Omar as one of the sort-of good guys? Even Barack Obama, when he was campaigning for the presidency in 2008, admitted that Omar was his favorite TV character.

"He's the toughest, baddest guy on the show," said Obama. "He's not my favorite person, but he's a fascinating character: a gay gangster who robs only drug dealers."

One way to look at it is to compare Omar with another of *The Wire*'s cold-blooded killers, Marlo Stanfield. There's a scene toward the end of the final season in Episode 4, when the rotund, east side drug boss, Proposition Joe, realizes that Marlo has betrayed him. Just before Joe is shot he complains, "I treated you like a son." Without a shred of sentiment, Marlo replies, "Wasn't meant to play the son."

Omar, in contrast, in Episode 7 of Season 1, wants to make sure Detective Bunk Moreland understands why he has given the police information that leads to the arrest of Marquis "Bird" Hilton for the murder of an ordinary citizen.

"I do some dirt too," says Omar, "but I never put my gun on nobody who wasn't in the game."

To which Bunk drily sighs, "A man must have a code."

Later, Omar testifies in court against Bird and has a testy exchange with defense attorney Maurice Levy. A crooked lawyer in the pay of the Barksdale organization, Levy gets Omar to admit that his occupation consists of robbing drug dealers. Levy, then, in a play to the jury, calls Omar a parasite.

"Just like you, man."

"Excuse me?" says Levy, whirling to face him, but falling right into Omar's trap.

"I got my shotgun," drawls Omar, "You got your briefcase."

The actor Michael Kenneth Williams, who portrayed Omar, once told ABC News: "People might not agree with his ethic or what he is about but they respect the fact he is honest. As they say in the 'hood, he's a stand-up kind of dude."

Clearly, Omar has a streak of the romantic in him that gives his character a sympathetic roundness approaching Robin Hood proportions. Meanwhile, Marlo's sociopathic, one-dimensional inhumanity seems like something out of a zombie movie.

Perhaps because Omar is human he doesn't realize that while his swagger and legend frighten away most players in his deadly street game, it has created an enemy out of a seemingly powerless nobody. In Episode 57, in *The Wire*'s final season, Omar is out to destroy as much of Marlo's drug trade as possible—in a ploy to get Marlo to come out and face him. He begins by killing Savino, one of Marlo's lieutenants. Limping from an injury incurred in an earlier close escape from Marlo, Omar then sneaks up on Michael Lee's drug corner. At gunpoint he steals Michael's drug stash and warns him to tell Marlo he is going to kill all of his people.

Watching this scene is twelve-year-old Kenard, one of Michael's corner hoppers. A smallish boy, Kenard bears the innocent face of a puppy but the bite and bark of a rabid pit bull. He appears to be homeless, certainly without parents, and every time he opens his mouth the words come out with a vicious, profane anger that belies his years. As Omar limps away from Michael, Kenard seems less than impressed at this first face-to-face with the great badman.

In the next episode, Omar is still at it, and this time he tips off two cops to the location of the drug stash of a group of Marlo's corner boys. Moving through the neighborhood, Omar comes on a handful of young boys who scatter in fear before him. All but one: Kenard.

Omar steps inside a corner grocery and is at the counter, purchasing his usual pack of Newports, when we hear the door to the grocery swing open. The next thing heard is a loud bang and Omar disappears from view. Kenard, holding an automatic pistol as big as his head, has come up behind him and shot Omar dead.

It is a thoroughly shocking moment. Longtime viewers of *The Wire* no doubt expected that Omar, at some point, would go down. But most likely that would happen in a raging gun battle with Marlo, and certainly with some choice Omarian words of street irony on his dying lips. Nobody saw it coming that the legendary Omar would be shot dead and speechless by a twelve-year-old boy.

PERHAPS IT'S THE PUBLIC HEALTH DOCTOR IN ME, but I had taken note since the first season of *The Wire* that very young kids like Kenard were acting with horrendous violence toward others, usually with guns. I'm not saying the show wasn't realistic. It was. David Simon and Ed Burns were reflecting the violence they knew too well from their years on the street. In fact, as Rafael Alvarez pointed out in his guide to *The Wire,* Burns years ago actually witnessed an Omar-like robber of drug dealers confronting a victim in a project courtyard. Concealed under a long "Jesse James duster coat" was a shotgun. From a stakeout location, says Alvarez, Burns watched as the man brought the shotgun out from beneath his coat and shot the drug dealer in the leg.

As some of us often do when watching a TV drama, I tend to mentally fill in the blanks behind a fictional character's motivation for an action, just to make sure it squares with what I know to be plausible. In a way it's a flight of fantasy, but a good script will lay enough groundwork to convince a viewer that the character's action was logical and made sense from a certain point of view.

When Omar went down, I added a pinch of real-life experience to my flight of fancy about the script writer's rationale behind Kenard's act. When I was health commissioner in Baltimore—even as scenes like this one were being played out on both the real and fictional streets of Baltimore—I dealt with an almost invisible problem that had very much to do with violence in and among children. That is why I began theorizing that while Omar certainly died from a lead bullet to the head, the real cause of his death could very well have been a killer more stealthy than Kenard: lead paint.

Civilizations have been mining lead for many thousands of years. In the nineteenth and twentieth centuries, it was used in gasoline to help lubricate an engine's valves, to make cans for food, and to increase the brightness and life of a coat of paint. Solder once contained lead as did the pipes that carried water inside our homes. Items such as crystal and ceramic pottery contained it and, because it has a sweet taste to it, ancient Romans even used lead in their wine making.

In the middle of the twentieth century, however, scientists made a startling discovery about houses with interiors covered in lead paint. Often, in poorly maintained older homes, chips of lead paint would flake to the floor and mingle with everyday dust. Throughout time, young children have crawled on these dusty floors and then, moments later, put their fingers in their mouths. If what they experienced was a sweet taste, those fingers very likely went back for more. The problem, some scientists found, was that those lead chips were highly toxic, a poison that was especially dangerous to very young children.

We now know that ingested lead affects neurological development—even those exposed to it in microscopic amounts. According to the Environmental Protection Agency (EPA), "it takes lead dust equal to two grains of sugar a day on a child's fingertip transferred to the mouth, for perhaps a month, to cause that child's nerve velocity to decrease, making the child slower both physically and mentally."

Lead paint poisoning mostly occurs in our older cities—on the east coast and in the Rust Belt, predominantly among children growing up in older, poorly maintained housing stock. Most lead poisoning occurs as a result of coming in contact with lead dust on floors, so babies and toddlers, who spend the most time crawling and playing on the floor, are the most likely to be exposed to this dust. Because a child's brain is developing rapidly at that age, the lead exposure is particularly damaging.

Not long after lead paint was banned in the United States in 1978, scientists began conducting long-range studies of the effects of exposure to lead, some of them following the same groups of children from birth into adulthood.

The first of those longitudinal studies was carried out in Cincinnati with children from the city's inner city neighborhoods where poverty had deep roots. Blood levels of the children in the study were measured even before birth, during their mother's pregnancy, and continuing for up to twenty-four years in some cases. Investigators for the Cincinnati Lead Study used magnetic resonance imaging, or MRI, to measure any changes in brain function over those years. They found that participants who showed high blood levels of lead as children showed "decreased gray matter" in their brains as adults.

Other researchers have connected childhood lead poisoning to violent behavior. In his 2008 article, Harvard professor David C. Bellinger, M.D., cites a study that links childhood lead poisoning to "arrests, since the age of 18 years, for violent offenses, drug offenses, theft or fraud, obstruction of justice, serious motor vehicle offenses, and disorderly conduct."

Dr. Bellinger, who is a professor of neurology in the Harvard Medical School and in the Harvard School of Public Health, also cites reports that connect lead poisoning with teen pregnancy, substance abuse, and attention-deficit hyperactivity disorder. He cautions that, even though the EPA guidelines suggested an alert level of 10 micrograms or more per deciliter of blood, a "safe" level has yet to be found. This was confirmed by a recent report from the Centers for Disease Control and Prevention that concluded that no amount of lead in the blood is safe. It is quite likely, though not easy to prove conclusively, that lead poisoning plays a significant role in the large number of students enrolled in special education programs in schools across the East and Midwest.

Similarly, Dr. Herbert Needleman of the University of Pittsburgh has found that "when environmental lead finds its way into the developing brain, it disturbs neural mechanisms responsible for regulation of impulse. That can lead to antisocial and criminal behavior."

In addition, researchers looking at the correlation between childhood lead exposure from leaded gas and violent behavior found that "the reduction in childhood lead exposure in the late 1970s and early 1980s was responsible for significant declines in violent crime in the 1990s and may cause further declines in the future."

Once poisoned, there is little effective treatment for youngsters. In fact, the only time medical treatment seems to be of value is when blood lead levels are so significantly elevated that serious acute physical problems, like seizures, coma, or death can occur. In those cases, heavy metals, called chelation agents, can be given intravenously to help remove lead from the blood. However, this is of no benefit for the much more common situation of lower level, long-term exposure to lead. Thus, the only recourse available for most lead poisoned kids is behavioral therapy to help children deal with the developmental or behavioral effects of this exposure.

HISTORICALLY, BALTIMORE PLAYED a key national role in addressing the problem of childhood lead poisoning. In the 1930s and the 1940s, Baltimore's longtime health commissioner, Dr. Huntington Williams, was the first major public health official in the country to raise awareness about the dangers of lead paint. There followed a ban of lead paint in Baltimore in 1950, long before the rest of the country caught on.

Unfortunately, the vast majority of the hundreds of thousands of houses and row houses built and painted before 1950 in Baltimore City—and especially those in the west Baltimore area where *The Wire* takes place—contain lead paint. Even those houses with new layers of unleaded paint still retain much of the original paint underneath, which perniciously releases the lead over time.

In the last couple of decades of the twentieth century far too little was done to deal with this problem, and the system of intervention that we did have was completely reactive, rather than proactive and preventive. The old system in Baltimore—which sounds impressive on paper—was supposed to work as follows: if a child was found to have an elevated blood lead level as a result of a visit to a pediatrician, the Baltimore City Health Department Childhood Lead Poisoning prevention program would be notified.

At that point, a health department environmental inspector would be sent to check the house for lead paint using a special x-ray machine

(XR-F) and, if lead paint was found, a violation notice would be sent to the property owner or landlord. Legally, the violation had to be abated within sixty days—and the affected child was to be moved out of the house until the lead problem was resolved. If the violation was not abated within that time period, the landlord was to be taken to court for enforcement action under the housing code. In addition to the inspectors, a nurse would be dispatched to ensure that the family was getting the appropriate care for the child.

There were significant problems with all aspects of this system. Thousands of young children never had blood tests because they didn't have a source of regular health care or, if they did have a doctor, the parent and that pediatrician lacked knowledge of the need to test for lead poisoning. In more than 75 percent of cases, inspectors did not gain access to the homes of children with elevated lead levels. Thus, violations were not issued in a timely manner, if at all. Violation notices, when generated, routinely sat untouched for weeks before being sent to landlords. By far the worst problem: not a single enforcement action was brought against a landlord in the entire decade of the 1990s.

The basic structure of the system was also flawed. Baltimore and other cities were essentially using children like "canaries in a coal mine"—to test whether houses had lead paint problems. This system of sporadically testing children after they might have been exposed, rather than proactively testing all houses where children lived to identify the problem before a poisoning occurred, clearly did not do enough to solve the problem.

During my tenure as commissioner, we radically revamped our entire approach to childhood lead paint poisoning. But it didn't happen all at once. As I was learning about and dealing with many major issues in my first few years as commissioner, due, in part, to the lack of good data on the problem, childhood lead poisoning simply didn't hit my radar screen. In addition, the lead poisoning program in the health department was the subject of a turf battle, with different components reporting to three separate assistant commissioners. Our deputy commissioner—whom I had replaced as commissioner—continued to lobby me not to change the system.

It took me some time before I realized the limitations of the existing approach. When I did, the reason for the lack of enforcement was obvious and simple: the cases had to be brought in housing court, but the housing commissioner at the time did not see lead cases as a priority. Thus we didn't get any of the precious docket time for our cases, and as a result, thousands of children in lead-infested properties suffered often irreversible lifelong neurologic and behavioral consequences, while scofflaw property owners were essentially held harmless.

All of this changed in early 2000. Shortly after Martin O'Malley took office as mayor, the Baltimore *Sun* ran a series of investigative stories that highlighted both the extent of the lead problem and the lack of a sensible system to address it. With this public prodding, the mayor proposed to Governor Parris Glendening that the state and city undertake a joint initiative to attack lead poisoning in Baltimore City. In the early spring Glendening and O'Malley publicly announced a new plan to be funded by $4.5 million per year added to the governor's 2001 budget.

BALTIMORE AND OTHER CITIES WERE ESSENTIALLY USING CHILDREN LIKE "CANARIES IN A COAL MINE"

The new lead initiative, run out of the city's department of health, was to be a collaborative effort between us, the city's department of housing and the state departments of health, housing, and environment. The United States Department of Housing and Urban Development and the Environmental Protection Agency were also paying close attention. Having had previous unsatisfactory experiences with interagency collaborations, I was more than a bit pessimistic about its prospects for success. But since the effort would be run and overseen by the health department, I had confidence in our ability to deliver. In fact, we mounted a huge effort comprising several strategies.

We immediately decided to hire a central coordinator to consolidate the oversight of all of the plan's parts. First on the agenda was developing an enforcement effort. Our coordinator hired two attorneys and set them loose on wayward landlords.

The fact that Baltimore property owners hadn't used lead paint since the 1950s was beside the point. It is an old city and, most of the houses had been painted with lead-based paint, and there weren't a lot of new houses being built. The issue became one of making sure property owners were taking steps to abate the existing problem, especially those renting properties in low income neighborhoods. Many were not—because they knew that the law wasn't being enforced, so they could act with impunity.

That changed dramatically when we launched our initiative in 2000, with the deputy housing commissioner, Denise Duval, prosecuting the first case against a city landlord in ten years. Within a year, we had filed more than 150 cases against property owners of addresses where a child had been poisoned. The first case that went to trial resulted in a judgment against the landlord for both money (a fine) and action (immediate lead abatement of the property). Over the next couple of years, another 550 cases were brought against miscreant landlords, and every one of them settled out of court in favor of the health department and the poisoned child. Landlords, both bad and mediocre, began to understand that the city was serious about addressing the problem, as the legal ground beneath them shifted dramatically.

What followed were a sizeable number of lead abatements by landlords on their own to clean up their properties. Because of legislation passed during this period at the state level, part of the requirement for abatement was that landlords conduct a full cleaning of a rental property in between tenants. Without it, a landlord would be prosecuted. We set up a LeadStat initiative—much like our KidStat and DrugStat programs—to track every property in question. When a house passed the cleaning inspection it went from red to green on our map. After the first landlord we prosecuted for failing to clean was found guilty, other property owners got the message. One after another, those red properties turned green.

Abatement isn't as easy as it may sound, even with landlord cooperation. Abatement of lead paint is a very expensive process because to do it right you first have to temporarily relocate a family from its home. Removing the paint and subsequent repainting could cost up to $20,000 per house. So we came up with a plan called "remediation," focusing primarily on heavily trafficked frictional surfaces within a home—such as windowsills and doorjambs, which generate the lead dust that ends up on the floor, where children are most likely to put their hands. To help those landlords and homeowners who couldn't afford to abate their properties, we started a grant program to help them. The process picked up after we put it entirely under the aegis of the city health department, rather than continuing to have it jointly administered with the housing department. We doubled the number of contractors who were certified to perform abatement work and quintupled the number of relocation homes where families were housed during the work. We also got payments out to contractors within three days of work being completed—virtually a miracle for a program run by city government. It was an accomplishment that ingratiated us with many contractors and property owners.

Along with our enforcement efforts, we started a major educational campaign aimed at parents and pediatric health care providers. We stressed the importance of testing all one- and two-year-olds in the city for lead. To help accomplish that goal, we introduced a piece of legislation in the city council (and companion legislation in the Maryland General Assembly) that required all children in this age group in zip codes with high levels of lead-painted houses to be given blood lead tests by their health care providers.

This sparked an unforeseen tussle with the Maryland Academy of Pediatricians over penalties that might be levied on doctors who didn't test their patients in a timely manner. The academy argued that the blame might better be placed on parents who didn't bring their children to the doctor in the first place. After assuring them that no penalties would be levied in the first year after enactment and that our intention was to work with and aid pediatricians in getting their patients in to see them on time, their opposition evaporated.

Both the city council and the General Assembly passed the bills into law. They have had a very beneficial effect—the percentage of one- and two-year-olds who got a blood lead test in Baltimore City increased 50 percent over the next two years to a level higher than any other jurisdiction in Maryland.

However, since research indicates that there is no such thing as a safe lead level in a very young child, our initiative took one step further. We launched the final phase of our initiative—early lead dust testing in the homes of pregnant women or newborn babies. This proactive approach actually won the top award from the U.S. Conference of Mayors, in 2002, as the most innovative and promising lead poisoning prevention strategy in the country. Under this project, all pregnant women and new mothers get a free lead dust test kit from their obstetrician, via our Childhood Lead Prevention Program, and are given instructions on how and where to test in their house for the presence of lead dust. Arrangements are then made to have the results relayed back in a short period of time. If high levels of lead are found, the problem can be abated before the baby arrives.

Put together, these three components of our lead initiative made a truly significant difference in the one statistic that really matters: the number of children with elevated lead levels in the city. Amazingly, even though we are testing many more one- and two-year-olds for lead now than prior to the initiative, the number of youngsters of those ages with elevated levels actually dropped by more than 80 percent in the decade after the program started: in 1999, 16.7 percent of children tested had blood levels of 10 micrograms per deciliter or above; a decade later, in 2009, that rate had dropped to less than 2 percent. Thus with a combination of preventive and proactive approaches, we were able to identify many lead-infested homes and abate the problem *before* a child became poisoned.

A child like Kenard, perhaps. For, whatever *The Wire*'s scriptwriters had in mind regarding Kenard's motivation in killing Omar, it struck me that his violent temper and aggression could easily be explained by an undiscovered case of lead poisoning as a very young child. In families that are poor and saddled with many stresses and challenges or in families where there is parental drug or other abuse, dysfunctional children like a Kenard or a Dukie or a Michael may never be tested for lead, even with a law on the books requiring exactly that. Unfortunately, these at-risk children are precisely the ones whom society can least afford to be further harmed by the scourge of lead poisoning. This is particularly true in light of the CDC's statement that there is no safe blood lead level in children. Thus, greater efforts must be made to eliminate this toxin from impoverished communities so that future Kenards can grow up without what is essentially a preventable form of brain damage.

Food choices are limited in many U.S. cities, one of the factors contributing to the escalating population of obese children and adults, including fix-it man Proposition Joe. In *The Wire*, this can be seen when bar food and booze, juice boxes and chips, and fried fish and candy crowd out healthy foods in the characters' daily diet. THE WIRE/HBO ©

CHAPTER 12

OBESE YET MALNOURISHED

THE WEIGHTY CONTRADICTION OF PROP JOE

SO, HOW MANY TIMES A WEEK do you think Kenard, the kid who shot Omar, or the real-life Corey from the Top of McKean Avenue Boys, sat down to a balanced dinner? Where does a child whose parents are addicts find something to eat on a daily basis? Often it's the corner store. Or think about poor Duquan—Dukie—whose parents are so irresponsible that they sell his clothes for drug money. There isn't enough money to buy food so Dukie can't pack a lunch. There isn't even cash for Dukie to buy junk food at the corner grocery. Mr. Prezbo, in Season 4, takes pity on him and gives him part of his own lunch.

The serious health issues that underlie the motivation of most characters from *The Wire* run the gamut from Bubs's heroin addiction and McNulty's unstated alcoholism to Tommy Carcetti's high stress and the homicide department's poor sleep habits. But it seems everybody on the show makes poor food choices, either out of necessity, ignorance, or a lack of self control.

It doesn't just show up in the obvious rotundity of certain characters like Sergeant Jay Landsman or Detective Bunk Moreland. Scene after scene depicts cops, corner boys, stevedores, lawyers, and others stuffing their faces with every variety of fast food. Randy Wagstaff secretly sells candy to his classmates; Omar walks across the street in his flowing silk bathrobe to get a box of sugar-coated cereal; Bodie and McNulty munch on fast-food burgers. Avon Barksdale is shown in prison eating smuggled-in Kentucky Fried chicken. And there is the young teenager, Wallace, acting as a parent for a houseful of small kids with no apparent families. He makes sure each child is dressed for school in the morning, then, as each goes out the door, he hands over a drink box and a bag of chips.

Over the past thirty or so years an epidemic of obesity has grown insidiously in the United States. The rate of obesity has quadrupled in children; a full 68 percent of adults are now overweight or obese, with the highest rate among low income individuals.

How did we get so fat? Partly, again, place matters. Neighborhoods without full-scale supermarkets (often called food deserts) are dominated by small corner convenience stores. The limited selection of snacks and sodas and grocery items in such stores are overpriced—the cost of convenience—and provide little in the way of the nutrition a body needs to function. Those already wise in the ways of nutrition understand that this is a serious issue, but for those who may lack a nutrition IQ, including many people who live in food deserts, the topic of vitamins and minerals may simply sound too boring or confusing to consider.

This is unfortunate, because, as a result of poor diet and a lack of exercise, the United States today is also in the midst of an epidemic of adolescent obesity. This epidemic has an impact on the lives of children of the inner city that can be as dangerous as the violence carried out by members of the Barksdale and Stanfield gangs. In fact, the poor food quality available contributes directly to childhood obesity in these neighborhoods. Consider that adults as obese as *The Wire*'s Proposition Joe likely started off as obese kids.

The lack of availability of healthy food and fresh produce in many neighborhoods was dramatically brought home to me one summer day at a café located at a city pool where my family and I were swimming. A young boy from a nearby impoverished community, who was probably twelve years old, had been hired by the owner to help her unload items she had bought at a farmer's market for the café. While I watched in disbelief, she asked the boy to go through the packages and get her some celery. He returned with a cucumber. After quietly correcting him, she asked him for a squash—only to have him bring back a radish. Why was he doing this? Because he had never seen these vegetables before in his life! The decreased availability of healthy food options in impoverished areas creates conditions that cause children from these neighborhoods to have some of the highest obesity rates in the country.

The ramifications of an unhealthy diet among inner city children are frightening: skyrocketing rates of chronic diseases in adolescents formerly seen almost exclusively in adults. Teens are developing type II diabetes—once known as adult-onset diabetes—at alarming rates, with the American Diabetes Association reporting that up to 45 percent of all cases diagnosed in this age group in 2000 were characterized as type II, up from less than 4 percent as recently as 1990. Indeed, by the late 2000s, almost one-quarter of all teens were diabetic or prediabetic, compared with less than 10 percent a decade earlier. Type II diabetes, caused by the degradation of the body's pancreatic function, is highly correlated with obesity and can lead to a whole host of bad health consequences down the road, including early stroke, heart disease, and blindness.

Similarly, hypertension, or high blood pressure, was rarely found in teens until recently. Also highly associated with obesity, this chronic condition puts its victims at far higher risk of early demise due to stroke and heart disease, among other things. In addition, teens are now showing signs of degenerative arthritis and other joint conditions that were almost never found in that age group in earlier generations. Due almost exclusively to excess weight, arthritis makes it even harder for overweight teens to exercise, even in moderation, thus consigning the young person to long-term weight problems. I clearly remember a fifteen-year-old girl at one of our school-based health centers who had severe degenerative arthritis in her knees caused by her extreme obesity.

One of the most disturbing findings in recent research on overweight children and teenagers is the high likelihood that excess weight in childhood leads to excess weight and obesity in adulthood: according to the American Academy of Child and Adolescent Psychiatry, obese children ages ten to thirteen have an 80 percent likelihood of being obese as adults. The long-term serious health consequences of excess weight and obesity for these individuals as adults are the same as for teens and include the following: hypertension, type II diabetes, stroke, heart disease, arthritis, gout, gallstones, sleep apnea, high-risk pregnancy, and increased risk of certain cancers.

In the United States in 2008, approximately 34 percent of all adults were characterized as overweight and another 34 percent as obese. Thus, more than two-thirds of all adults had a significant weight problem. In contrast, during the 1960s 31 percent of American adults were categorized as overweight and only 13 percent were obese.

Even more alarming are statistics from a study of fourteen thousand individuals published in the *Journal of the American Medical Association* that clearly showed that obesity by age twenty leads to a significantly reduced life span. For those seriously obese at age twenty, defined as having a body mass index (BMI) greater than 45 (representative of this BMI is a man who is 6 feet tall and 330 pounds or a woman who is 5 feet, 4 inches, and 230 pounds), white men lose thirteen years of life, black men twenty years, white women eight years, and black women five years.

THE ECONOMIC COSTS OF OBESITY are staggering—best estimates are that direct and indirect costs are in the range of $150 billion per year. We will have a significantly less productive workforce if too many of our citizens suffer from chronic debilitating conditions secondary to being overweight. Our armed forces are even having a problem finding enough healthy individuals to serve in the military because these behaviors and conditions are so prevalent in our society today.

Public policy relating to our youngsters hasn't helped the situation, either. In many places, physical education requirements are virtually non-existent. In Maryland, for example, only one semester of physical education is required for high school students during their entire four years. Across the country, only one out of five high school seniors takes physical education classes. All of this at a time when we have seen a precipitous decline in physical activity as a part of everyday life. For example, half of all children walked to school in 1969, but only about one in ten do so today. Compounding the problem, on the nutrition side, many cash-strapped public schools have contracted with snack companies to install vending machines, which generate revenue, a portion of which goes to the schools. Unfortunately, many kids buy the unhealthy foods stocked in these machines, foods that usually contain very high fat and sugar content and have just empty, non-nutritional calories.

How can we combat the large societal trends of consumption of fast foods, advertisements for which permeate the airwaves, and the lack of physical activity? At least for kids, a couple of simple school policy changes could make a big difference.

First, local jurisdictions should mandate that all students—kindergarten through twelfth grade—be required to participate in either a physical education course or an extracurricular physical activity (such as athletic teams or dance) every semester. It would also be helpful if elementary schools ensured that kids have time and space to run around during recess—increasingly limited in many schools, as recess times are severely truncated or eliminated. This time of free play does wonders for relieving pent-up energy in young children as well as providing much-needed physical activity.

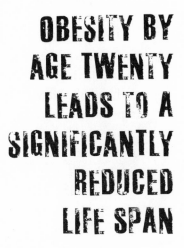

OBESITY BY AGE TWENTY LEADS TO A SIGNIFICANTLY REDUCED LIFE SPAN

Another needed school policy change involves increasing the availability of healthier food choices. We should eliminate candy and soda from vending machines in all schools—something currently proposed in several locales around the country. Although vending machines can be important sources of revenue, a simultaneous effort to educate kids on healthier snack and drink choices may be necessary to create similar demand for healthier products in alternative vending machines. Then, school cafeterias must offer healthy and nutritious food choices, from locally grown produce (as is done in several school districts in California) to healthy entrée alternatives like fresh fish and veggie burgers rather than hot dogs and fried chicken.

In reality, since so many of the eating behaviors of kids and adults are influenced by societal trends and the mass media, only so much can be done at the school level. There must be a concerted effort by public health advocates, pediatricians and other health care providers, government officials, and educators to let the public know how important a sensible diet is to the overall health and well-being of our country.

Combating the messages of big money food conglomerates will not be easy. For every public service announcement that health advocates could place, there will be dozens of commercials for the most popular fast-food burger franchises. But, just as anti-tobacco ads eventually got the message across—aided, of course, by an agreement to cease television and radio tobacco product ads—so, too might anti–fast-food ads and public service announcements.

Unfortunately, creating a public health message to combat the obesity epidemic is more difficult than dealing with the consequences of smoking or driving without seat belts. In those cases, the messages aimed at the public were crystal clear: don't smoke and you will dramatically improve your current and future health; wear seat belts and—if you get into an accident—you are much more likely to survive. These campaigns proved tremendously successful at decreasing smoking and increasing seat belt use.

In contrast, dietary messages are numerous—and often contradictory: "Eat a pack-of-cards size helping of meat each day" versus "go meat-free"; or "get on a no carb diet" versus "eat plenty of complex carbs"; "eat several small meals a day" versus "eat three well-balanced meals a day, including a healthy breakfast." It goes on and on and on. The plentitude of messages makes most people just throw their hands up in frustration.

That's why our health department in Howard County, Maryland (where I am now the health director), is trying a new tack: let's try to address the biggest single cause of weight gain, rather than attempt to tackle the totality of all sources of obesity. To that end, research clearly shows that the biggest single cause of excess calories in Americans' diets is the consumption of sugar-sweetened beverages, from sodas to sugar-filled "juice" drinks to energy drinks. Drawing from this research, we decided to focus our messaging on sodas—the epitome of empty calories. In 2011 we launched a soda-free pledge throughout the county, with the idea being that even cutting soda consumption by half would make a serious dent in an individual's daily calorie intake.

Of course, pledges and press conferences alone will not change attitudes and behaviors, but a consistent message from multiple sources may well have an effect on Americans' habits—just as consistent, singular messages affected smoking and seat belt usage. Even with this extra, specific focus on sodas, however, healthy eating habits must be encouraged at school and at home.

If we don't mount these comprehensive, community-based efforts, ultimately, those most susceptible to the pressure of fast-food advertisements and the lure of cheap, fast-food restaurants will continue to be inner-city youngsters and adults who have higher rates of obesity and are overweight in general. In other words, just by living where he does, Prop Joe faces a much greater likelihood of suffering from serious and debilitating chronic diseases than someone living in a less impoverished area, as well as a reduced life expectancy. Without significant changes in the food environment, he and many like him in real-world America will be consigned to a lifetime of being overweight yet undernourished.

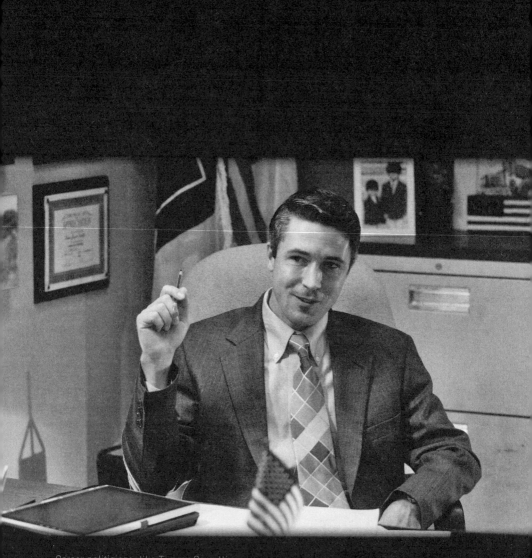

Career politicians, like Tommy Carcetti on *The Wire*, often start off with the purest of motivations to address public health issues and other systemic problems. Real-life situations often force them to rethink their approach, sometimes benefitting citizens and sometimes ignoring their needs. THE WIRE/HBO ©

CHAPTER 13

PUBLIC HEALTH AND POLITICS

THE PROMISE AND PERIL OF TOMMY CARCETTI

THE WHEELING AND DEALING OF POLITICS underlies every facet of life through the sixty episodes of *The Wire*. It measures the shifting balance of power from the judiciary, the police, city and state politics, the school administration, the fading working class on the waterfront, and even in the machinations of drug-dealing organizations.

Politics is supposed to be the art of the possible, but watching *The Wire* makes one think that perhaps it should be called the threat to the possible. For it's easy to come away from this series with the pessimistic feeling that the world is controlled by base political motives.

Indeed, just as *The Wire* is an indictment of public institutions in Baltimore (and everywhere, for that matter), it also exposes the failure of political discourse in the real world on numerous levels. As graphically portrayed week after week, those failures have helped a sizeable percentage of real-life Baltimore citizens to live, at the very least, less productive lives than they might have and, at worst, to see their lives slide into disaster.

- The city police department constantly takes the political pulse before almost any wheel turns—from shifting responsibility for solving murders to cooking statistics to show that crime has fallen when it has not.

- On the waterfront, in the second season, union boss Frank Sobotka takes payoffs from drug kingpins to help bring the scourge of heroin into the city aboard container ships. Why? In the perverse hope that he can hire lobbyists to bribe legislators to pass legislation that will bring work back to the docks.

- In the fourth season, set mostly in a city middle school, teachers are told that the most important thing is not educating children but making the school administration look good by raising test scores.

- In episodes that deal with public politics itself, the white, win-at-all-costs Tommy Carcetti is elected mayor in a predominantly black city because he cynically burns a friendship with a black colleague to split the minority vote. Ultimately, Carcetti wins the all-important support of the city's extensive network of black pastors—with backroom deals rooted in cynicism and self-interest.

- Even in the drug world, political chicanery takes place behind the scenes. Stringer Bell tries to wrest control of Avon Barksdale's drug organization by paying off a corrupt state senator to pull the right strings so his development project succeeds. In fact, State Senator Clay Davis double-crosses Bell, keeps the bribe money—and pulls no strings.

- Meanwhile, in the city's other major drug kingdom, Proposition Joe's political style is all about dialogue: eliminating jealousy and cultivating peace among rival gangs so that everyone in the drug business makes more money off the poor and vulnerable and stays alive. However, the intrusive politics of one of those rivals, Marlo Stanfield, are less complicated. Basically, if people disagree with you, kill them.

The Wire often casts political maneuvering as a bludgeon used by corrupt or amoral power brokers to thwart moral and civil justice while maximizing their own interests. This, even as the quality of education, policing, city services—even the purity of the heroin sold to desperate addicts—deteriorates.

And yet, to anyone sincerely interested in changing public policies regarding our health and safety, politics needs to be engaged at a level where it is still the honorable art of the possible. To be an effective proponent of public health one must not only have worthwhile ideas but also be able to translate those ideas into action with what many in the health arena consider distasteful tools: politics and money. Yet, the basic truth is that bringing ideas to reality requires money. To raise funds, to go after money, one must to be able to play the game of politics. Perhaps, though, "play" and "game" are the wrong terms. To accept politics as a valuable and honorable pursuit, one must take it seriously enough to *practice it*, just as a professional would practice medicine or law.

> **THE WIRE EXPOSES THE FAILURE OF POLITICAL DISCOURSE IN THE REAL WORLD ON NUMEROUS LEVELS**

What is the alternative? To be an effective policy advocate one cannot deal with issues in an academic vacuum. Simply debating policy implications with colleagues doesn't get the job done, no matter how promising or useful the idea may be. Without political support, nothing will happen. To have an impact on public policy requires a willingness to move within the political system and knowing who the legislators are in whatever jurisdiction you hope to exert influence and then knowing what buttons to push to get their attention and support.

One of the harsh realities exposed on *The Wire* is that there are not a lot of terribly caring or thoughtful politicians out there. To succeed, you still have to convince them that your mission is both feasible and worthwhile. In Baltimore we were able to get a law modified so we could set up a needle exchange. The politicians who controlled the votes to make that happen were not scientists or health professionals, but we were able to appeal to their interests, whether economic, issue driven, or purely political.

That doesn't mean we ignored the science. Indeed, we brought experts in to brief legislators on the science behind the AIDS epidemic. We didn't, however, depend on science alone. Basically, needle exchange was a political win. As noted in chapter 5, we put such pressure on the governor that he'd have had to arrest a black mayor and a white health commissioner to stop us from creating a needle exchange without his support. And at the same time, we were getting legislative support by presenting politically palatable ways for people to vote for it.

GIVEN THE CORRUPT BRAND OF POLITICS portrayed on *The Wire*, there are a few solid examples of characters grasping the moral distortions and perils of a situation and succeeding—with integrity still intact.

Look at the case of Cedric Daniels, who is a lieutenant when we first meet him. Somewhere in his past, we are led to believe, Daniels did something he wasn't proud of—most likely accepting some kind of low level payoffs in his days as a precinct cop. He has emerged unscathed from those days (although not completely, we are later to learn) and seems to have recognized the error of his old ways. He is determined to play it straight.

But when he steps into his first scene in *The Wire*, heading an ad hoc narcotics squad looking into Avon Barksdale's gang—his rule is tentative and conservative. That sparks conflict with Detective McNulty, who has a uniquely aggressive approach.

Daniels soon understands that he is expected by top police brass to make quick, cosmetic arrests of Avon Barksdale's low level drug dealers and then move on to something else. What the top brass wanted were arrests and "drugs on the table," and with them the kind of positive publicity that will support Mayor Clarence Royce in his reelection campaign (and keep their own careers on track). But Daniels refuses, keeping the case against Barksdale going full bore. Colonel Rawls threatens Daniels, but he goes over Rawls's head and appeals directly to Police Commissioner Burrell for more time on the case—which by that time was very effectively using a wiretap.

Burrell agrees and gives him more time. But, then, under increasing political pressure on himself, Burrell threatens to expose Daniels's past if his squad doesn't make arrests *now*—even though they don't have enough evidence to send Barksdale away for a long time. Daniels is defiant, but the arrests go down. Barksdale and several members of his gang get short prison sentences. On paper, a victory, but as usual in the War on Drugs, the big fish get away, largely untouched. In the next four seasons, Daniels faces more political pressure to manipulate crime statistics. He maintains his integrity through a grasp of the political system in both the police department and city hall. Through a series of political crises—some of them wins, some of them defeats—Daniels eventually rises to become police commissioner himself. But in the final season's last episode he is told by the staff of Mayor Carcetti, now running for governor, to make it look like crime has fallen by 10 percent. If Daniels refuses, information about his past will be made public. Recognizing he has gone as far as he can politically without selling his soul, Daniels resigns rather than give in. Although he doesn't "win" in the sense of achieving his policy goal, the lesson is that by figuring out the politics without compromising his ethics and sticking to his own moral code, Daniels furthers his goal as far as he can, with the possibility of returning to fight another day. In the end, he chooses integrity over power. Viewers can learn from his example as well as from those of many other "politicians" on *The Wire* who found the temptation of power too alluring to resist.

Certainly, Commissioner Burrell and Mayor Royce fit the definition of political hacks who were always in it for their own gain. Their duplicity wasn't as shocking, perhaps, as that of the fictional Baltimore *Sun* reporter Scott Templeton, the character who invented facts to make his stories more powerful—eventually winning a Pulitzer Prize for his sins. Or even our heroic/antiheroic McNulty, a character whose morals may have been down there around slim and none but whose ethics as a police detective always seemed rock solid. In the end, he stoops to creating a phony serial killer case to win more time for detectives to gain evidence against Marlo Stanfield.

And let us not forget Bunny Colvin, the police major caught in a political crossfire caused partly by his own actions, but in a larger part by the political cynicism of his superiors. Colvin's decision to create what turned into Hamsterdam—that creative, though impossible, arrest-free zone of drug dealers far from harm's way—was noble, if politically naive. At least Colvin had the good of the city on his mind, whereas his bosses had personal advancement on theirs. Like Daniels, Colvin's story didn't turn out successfully, at least with respect to his career. But the two men clearly emerged in the sadder-but-wiser category and with their self-respect intact.

I've long felt that the reason for seeking office, whether in the state legislature, or city hall, or Congress, is to make a difference. You have to know going in what you are and are not willing to do to hold that office. That means you need to be willing, up front, to be a one term councilman or mayor or whatever. Because the trappings of the position—even for city council members, who can delude themselves into thinking they are someone special—make public office so attractive, one may otherwise be tempted to compromise too much in order to avoid giving it up.

In my experience in Maryland politics, I've run into a select few truly courageous legislators. The one who first comes to mind is Ron Guns, a very conservative Democrat from rural Cecil County in northeastern Maryland. In 1994 he was chair of the Environmental Matters Committee in the Maryland House of Delegates. He took the lead role in advocating for a needle exchange on our behalf at great political peril to his career. He did this solely because he felt it was a potentially life-saving initiative and the right thing to do. I give him huge credit for that. I can think of other legislators who often take principled positions, but none who have acted as courageously.

In any system, there will be politics, particularly in government circles where the lingua franca is politics. The two highest ranking politicians I worked for in Baltimore were mayors Kurt Schmoke and Martin O'Malley. Both Democrats, their styles and motivations in governing were completely different—something I had to adjust to if I was to have any hope of moving the policies of the health department forward. I think one of my greatest challenges was in finding politically acceptable ways to do just that.

Schmoke was very cause oriented. An intellectual with a humanitarian bent, he saw the importance of needle exchange because it made sense in terms of reducing AIDS. It appealed to him because people were dying unnecessarily. Schmoke spent a lot of time thinking through all sides of an issue, particularly how a proposal would affect individual citizens. As he thought about how to piece the puzzle together, he started addressing some deep-seated problems like education reform and medicalizing the drug issue. He was way ahead of his time.

Unfortunately his administration did a relatively poor job of publicizing his successes, so that most of the publicity he got came when things went wrong. He was a much more successful mayor than people give him credit for. He took on the big issues with no easy solutions, yet he was able to affect the debate on many of them, including drug policy, at the national level. It wasn't a big blow for Schmoke's ego when he stepped down as mayor. He could take it or leave it.

His successor, in contrast, was a publicity savvy, charismatic politician who was driven to lead and had ambitions of a long political career. When you have someone like that becoming mayor of a city, there's going to be a balancing act between political motivations and an even-handed approach to decision making.

O'Malley had essentially two things on his political agenda as mayor. One: show he could manage the city well. At that he was quite successful. Second: get crime down, particularly homicides. Everything was focused on that. This is why he vigorously supported increased funding for drug treatment. It wasn't because he was convinced that the War on Drugs was a failure and immoral, but because getting people treatment and off drugs would likely reduce crime and thus made sense for his crime policy. Therefore, on a variety of fronts, in order for my public health agenda to be successful I had to make it dovetail with his agenda—and his agenda included being elected to higher office in the future.

A perfect example was Operation Safe Kids. O'Malley asked me to lead a group of officials to analyze why juvenile homicides had spiked in 2001. We came back with a proposal to implement the Operation Safe Kids program described in chapter 1. We pitched it, in part, as a crime prevention effort and a way to get the ignominious distinction of the city with the worst juvenile violence rate in the country off our back. Had we not framed our issues to fit his agenda, the public health benefits of this policy would never have occurred. Similarly, while we pushed drug treatment for the humanitarian benefit it would provide to addicted individuals and their families, that was not nearly as appealing to O'Malley as the effect it would have on reducing crime. By working in concert with the mayor, we were able to achieve his goals as well as our own.

Politics has always been a somewhat invisible force behind the implementation of any public policy strategy. Still in an earlier, less contentious political climate, the enactment of public health measures was seldom questioned. Part of the reason, undoubtedly, is that measures such as clean water and eradication of disease just seemed so logical and patently beneficial to all. Consider that in the mid-1950s, hundreds of thousands of schoolchildren were vaccinated with an unproven, anti-polio virus developed by the virologist Jonas Salk. The public fear of polio was so great then that the vaccine trials went forward with very little public protest.

IN AN EARLIER, LESS CONTENTIOUS POLITICAL CLIMATE, THE ENACTMENT OF PUBLIC HEALTH MEASURES WAS SELDOM QUESTIONED

Public health policy is no longer so clear cut and the politics behind today's strategies are more complicated than in the past. Arguing against reason that drug addiction is a crime that must be punished, and not a disease that ought to be treated, has become a very common and visible campaign issue for many would-be office holders. If I say drug addicts aren't criminals, it is argued, then the public will perceive me as weak and they will not elect me.

Neither the show *The Wire* nor this book will easily change attitudes so deeply and so wrongly held. Not necessarily felt, but held, and there's a distinction between the two. One of the peculiar idiosyncrasies of language that emerged from *The Wire*—along with street-level slang such as "true dat" and "most def"—is a simple question often posed by Omar in the middle of a conversation. When he asks, "You feel me?" Omar isn't wondering if he has been heard. Rather he seeks understanding at the profound level of kinship, one that is recognized by members of the same tribe. Whenever Omar asked that question, I always got the impression that the tribe he had in mind was all encompassing. It included everyone. Not just Butchie or Bunk or drug dealers or blacks or whites. Perhaps that is why the character of Omar is so hard to pigeonhole or stereotype. That's because Omar is painted with a rich and full palette. Omar is real and we do feel him.

The ultimate politics of *The Wire*, the real politics that goes to the heart as well as the mind, is the simple and complicated influence of people upon people. If we are honest with ourselves, we can not only see the truth in the various scenes and characterizations invented for us by the writers and directors, but we can feel those people as people. Why then can't we get up from our televisions and look through our windows and see and feel the world going on around us the same way? Is it because of attitudes deeply and wrongly held?

In the end, the value of *The Wire*, I think, is that it makes one want to dig deeper, all the way down to that Omar level of feeling. Because down there at that level is where real change is born.

Selected for a pilot program to help
children who cannot function in regular
classrooms. Namond Brice's life turns
around after meeting Howard "Bunny"
Colvin and social work professor David
Parenti. Place matters, but so does the
dedication of those striving to better
the lives of pawns in the drug war.
THE WIRE/HBO ©

LEARNING FROM THE WIRE

PRACTICING POLITICS TO PRACTICE MEDICINE

FREQUENTLY CALLED THE SECOND OLDEST profession, many people regard politics as a cynical game and politicians as self-interested individuals who are looking to make a buck and who are most certainly not out to serve the public good. Although this view has some merit, throughout history many of humankind's greatest achievements have been attained through the noble practice of politics, which, simply put, is a means for a diverse community to find consensus as it attempts to solve its problems. With an emphasis on finding consensus, practicing politics becomes the worthy pursuit of creating a better life.

During the first years of the new millennium, we began to consider a broader goal that would benefit not just Baltimore residents but all Americans' quality of life: assuring health care for all. Indeed, pushing for health care reform became not only the biggest challenge I had faced thus far but one that took every bit of the political training and capital I had accumulated through years of trial and error. Developing grassroots coalitions, knowing how to appeal to individual politicians, devising a mass communication strategy for a complex subject, and figuring out how to deal with well-financed special interests—these were critical skills for anyone who hoped to reform an inequitable, complicated, and far too expensive system that had become broken. In fact, I believe that fixing our health care system would help ameliorate many of the problems portrayed in *The Wire.*

It had become increasingly evident in those years that far too much of our political and financial capital was being spent on dealing with the problems of the uninsured and underinsured in a piecemeal fashion. As an example, immense political effort had been made by Mayor Schmoke, myself, and large numbers of advocates for increased funding for substance abuse treatment. What many in the general public—and I think in the state legislature as well—failed to understand at the time, was that the funding was for *uninsured* substance users. Those with insurance who had a substance abuse problem generally had coverage for treatment and didn't need public funding.

UNINSURED AMERICANS ARE SICKER, AND DIE EARLIER, THAN THOSE WHO HAVE INSURANCE

Similar efforts had been undertaken to fund breast and cervical cancer screening and mental health services—again for the uninsured. This Band-Aid approach struck me as both inefficient and unproductive. It pushed me to begin working on a much more humane and sensible plan to provide comprehensive health coverage for everyone in Maryland.

The need for it in Maryland and nationwide is hard to deny. Currently about 52 million Americans have no health coverage and an additional 25 million are underinsured, defined as those who can't afford basic primary and preventive care because of high deductibles or copayments. Thus, in any given year more than one in four Americans has either no or inadequate health insurance. To me, this lack of coverage is unconscionable in the wealthiest, most technologically advanced country in the world.

The uninsured are much more likely than those with insurance to go without regular checkups and other preventive services, including potentially life-saving screening tests. They are much less likely to get care for chronic diseases such as hypertension, diabetes, heart disease, and arthritis. Therefore, those without insurance are much more likely to be hospitalized for, or die from, a condition that could have been avoided.

Ironically, the health services that the uninsured do obtain, often through emergency rooms, end up costing more than the same services provided to an insured individual. This is because most insurance plans, along with government programs like Medicare and Medicaid, negotiate large discounts with health care providers and hospitals. Those discounts are not available to the uninsured. Because of that, many uninsured often have to make a choice between medical care and other necessities of life, like food or shelter.

In our incredibly affluent country, with all of its advanced medical technology and services, tens of millions of our fellow citizens are effectively denied access to much of our world class medical system. What this all adds up to is this: uninsured Americans are sicker, and die earlier, than those who have insurance.

In the spring of 1998, I invited a small number of progressive colleagues to my office to look into the possibility of launching a universal health coverage initiative in Maryland. After a spirited discussion, we adjourned with each colleague's mandate to invite ten more interested individuals to the next meeting. After similar meetings over the next two months, our group had grown into a coalition of several hundred supporters. We eventually moved our gatherings to the larger state medical society headquarters.

After a few months, it became clear to me that we needed an actual organization with full-time staff to have any realistic chance of developing a Maryland health coverage initiative that could win broad-based community support. For that job we hired Vincent DeMarco, a savvy political veteran who had succeeded in getting several progressive social policies enacted in Maryland through shrewd use of the political process. He'd headed a coalition that passed a voter referendum banning Saturday night special guns and other weapons in Maryland and, at the time—the spring of 1999—was just finishing the successful effort to get the Maryland General Assembly to pass the only tobacco tax increase in the nation that year, in order to decrease teen tobacco use.

DeMarco and I made the rounds of local foundations looking for start-up money. Bob Embry of the Abell Foundation came through as usual, and within a couple of months, the Maryland Citizens' Health Initiative was born. DeMarco was the executive director, and I served as president. We formed a board, made up of a diverse group of individuals—church leaders, union leaders, public health professionals, and concerned citizens. This important preliminary work done, we then embarked on a two-part strategy.

First, we set out to develop that broad-based coalition of supporters. The need for grassroots support was one of the lessons we learned from the debacle of the Clinton health reform proposal of the early 1990s. A complete lack of any grassroots groundwork consigned their plan to a fiery death at the hands of large corporate interests, mainly in the insurance industry, who mounted an effective populist ad campaign.

We wrote a "Declaration of Health Care Independence" that included our bedrock values: universality, comprehensiveness, quality, and affordability. Over the next couple of years that declaration served as the most important grassroots organizing piece in recruiting organizations willing to join our campaign.

We went after organizations rather than individuals for a couple of reasons. Organizational support is often more impressive to legislators. And we could use the information-disseminating structures of various organizations to get our message out to more individuals than we could reach on our own.

Through an immense amount of work over many months, we enlisted 2,300 organizations, large and small. They included almost every statewide religious institution; physician, nursing, and social work groups; community associations; businesses and unions; and city and county councils. We became the largest coalition on any issue in Maryland history. We also held a series of community forums in every part of the state in which we presented our goals and ideas for a reformed system and listened to individual concerns. The forums provided us with useful input for devising a final plan and also gave thousands of citizens a sense of inclusion.

The second element of our two-part strategy was drafting proposed legislation. We had developed relationships with respected health policy, health economics, and health law experts from the University of Maryland, the Johns Hopkins University Bloomberg School of Public Health, and Georgetown University.

Initially, we supported a single-payer approach as the most equitable and cost-efficient proposal. In such a system—similar to that used in Canada and many other countries—all payment for health services comes from a single payer (generally the government) to health care providers and hospitals. The amount of payment is negotiated in advance by the single-payer entity and by the provider or hospital groups.

In a single-payer system, health care coverage is generally quite comprehensive, with low administrative costs since the "middle men"—insurance companies—are eliminated.

Early on, however, it became apparent that a single-payer system was politically problematic, and, if that was what we proposed, our plan would be dead on arrival. The opposition actually came from all sides. Union leaders—among the strongest backers of our initiative—didn't want a single-payer proposal because so much of their past efforts had been devoted to securing better health benefits for their members. A single-payer proposal would undercut one of their primary roles. Many in our support base of organizations feared that their members would be forced to abandon their current health coverage—which they considered to be good—in exchange for something new and unproven, no matter how good it sounded.

Meanwhile, the political right attacked us as socialists and communists (a preview of their response a decade later to health care reform legislation proposed by President Barack Obama). Insurance brokers argued that a single-payer plan would put them out of business regardless of how beneficial it would be for the state's citizens. The mammoth pharmaceutical industry weighed in, declaring the plan both socialistic and damaging to the future of medical research. Others argued that a single-payer plan in Maryland would result in higher taxes and would force many businesses to flee the state.

Most of those attacks, misleading at best and flat out wrong at worst, were relatively easy to counter. But because there were so many groups of so many stripes arrayed against a single-payer proposal, it seemed more sensible, politically, to look into other options. In the course of planning our legislation, we spent hundreds of hours strategizing with our consultants and meeting with every conceivable stakeholder to ascertain their views on the current health care system and how best to achieve universal coverage. We met with pediatricians, nurses, unions, insurance agents, small business owners, advocates for the disabled, legislators, and more. Sometimes those stakeholders would arrive for a meeting with us only to come face to face with an archenemy who was just leaving.

Even so, those meetings gave stakeholders from both sides some assurance that their views were being heard. A side benefit was the political cover the meetings gave in the event we were later asked if we had talked to such and such a group. We talked to everyone, and, in the process, found dozens of useful ideas for inclusion in our proposed legislation.

While work on the new proposal continued, we prepared for the 2002 Maryland elections—a time when every legislative seat and the governor's office would be up for grabs. Maryland is one of the most heavily Democratic states in the country. It had reliably supported the Democratic nominee in all presidential elections in the past two decades and consistently elected a Democrat to the governor's office and a huge Democratic majority to the House of Delegates and State Senate. In many legislative districts, the Democratic primary was the decisive election.

In September of 2002, two months ahead of the general election, we set out to get as many candidates as possible, both Democratic and Republican, to sign a pledge to support major components of our universal coverage plan. This had been a part of our general grassroots concept from the beginning and was based on a successful strategy used by DeMarco in prior issue-oriented initiatives.

With one rather glaring exception, our efforts during that election season were a resounding success. Seventy of those soon-to-be seated in the House of Delegates signed the pledge to support the major components of our plan. We were just one vote short of a majority of the 141-member chamber. In the Senate we had eighteen pledges, including three of the four committee chairs. We were only a handful of votes short of a majority in the forty-seven-member upper chamber. Those numbers gave us confidence we'd be able to obtain the support of the few additional legislators needed to make a majority.

But what we didn't count on was the first Republican victory for governor since Spiro Agnew's upset win thirty-six years before. Most member organizations in our coalition had supported the Democratic nominee for governor, Kathleen Kennedy Townsend—Bobby Kennedy's daughter—over the Republican, Congressman Robert Ehrlich.

Townsend supported our initiative, but Ehrlich was openly dismissive of it. During the summer, even though Townsend held a surprisingly small lead in the polls, Ehrlich's opposition was of only modest concern. Only in the last two weeks of the campaign did we increasingly realize that the likelihood of our success in Annapolis in the near future was about to drop dramatically. Unfortunately, our executive director, Vincent DeMarco, was a longtime thorn in Ehrlich's side, having run issue-oriented ads against him in a variety of campaigns, including—most painfully for us—this one. In addition, most of the major players and groups supporting the new governor in his election were not, to put it mildly, big fans of our initiative.

BELIEVERS IN POLITICS AS THE ART OF THE POSSIBLE SHOULD NOT FORGET THE LESSONS OF *THE WIRE*

In the months before the election, our new plan—again, without the single-payer structure—began to emerge. Although still true to our initial Declaration of Health Care Independence goals of four years prior—universality, affordability, quality, and comprehensiveness—the new proposal was intentionally cast in "conservative-friendly" language. It was basically a market-based public-private partnership for universal coverage (not much different at all from the Obama health reform bill passed in 2010). Utilizing four major sources of health coverage—three already existing (Medicaid, Medicare, and employer-sponsored health coverage with a small, new "public option"), this plan was easy to explain to the public. It did not require massive new public outlays and was much less threatening to a variety of business interests.

Our long and intense campaign didn't achieve what we had hoped, though it did allow me and thousands of dedicated supporters a chance to be heard on one of the most important issues of our day. My only regret is surrendering the single-payer option without a fight. It is a decision I regret to this day, as the problems with implementation of some of the parts of President Obama's health care reform act become increasingly evident.

Fortunately in politics, if you don't burn too many bridges, you have a chance to fight another day. That chance, the opportunity to design a much better system of care, would avail itself in the very same Obama health care reform legislation—section 1322 of the Affordable Care Act (ACA), to be precise. This little-known part of the act enables the formation of nonprofit health insurance cooperatives (CO-OPs).

As soon as the act was signed by President Obama in late March 2010, we put together a group of interested parties throughout Maryland to work on the development of such a CO-OP, both because it allowed for the creation of an innovative health care delivery system, and because it allowed us to target a population—working-class families and individuals— that would still have great difficulty affording health coverage even after the president's health care reforms took full effect. By way of example, a family of four making about $66,000 per year, or 300 percent of the federal poverty level, even with federal affordability subsidies, will still have to pay at least $6,500 after taxes for their premium alone. Either that, or forgo coverage and pay more than $2,000 in tax penalties for not complying with the individual mandate that virtually everyone must obtain coverage— thus, a serious financial dilemma for most working-class families.

To address this problem, our group set out to design a more affordable system of health care, while prioritizing primary and preventive care. Our CO-OP model is based on three pillars:

1. A primary care home model—where the vast majority of all care is provided at the primary care provider's office (including video consults with specialists)

2. Payment reform—all our providers will be salaried, getting rid of all fee-for-service payments, which have the perverse incentive of encouraging providers to prescribe unnecessary tests or procedures as each brings in revenue

3. Evidence-based medicine—where our providers will follow protocols for the most effective treatments and medications proven by research

Our actuarial studies have predicted that this combination of principles will result in insurance policies costing about a third less than conventional private insurance. Thus, it is our hope that not only will we be providing high quality care to our members, when the CO-OP is launched in 2014, but also that it will be affordable for those who might otherwise have had to go without insurance.

In the meantime, and in terms of changing policy on other vital issues that affect the public's health, believers in politics as the art of the possible should not forget the lessons of *The Wire*. The series never set out as a crusade for drug treatment, or a repurposing of criminal justice funding, or a more honest understanding of addiction and poverty. Its purpose was to tell a story, and it did that very well. Ironically, with all of its fictional devices and characters, it turned out to be a story almost too real to believe. Almost. That's why it succeeded, because we did believe what we saw. And in such belief lie the seeds of action.

CAST OF CHARACTERS

This list contains only those characters from *The Wire* mentioned in this book. For information on characters not included here, see www.hbo.org /the-wire.

THE GANG MEMBERS

Avon Barksdale, Baltimore drug lord

Bernard, part of Avon Barksdale's drug organization

Brother Mouzone, hired gun and enforcer from New York

"Butchie," blind restaurant owner and confidante of Omar Little

Calvin "Cheese" Wagstaff, nephew of "Prop" Joe and later part of Marlo Stanfield's drug organization

Chris Partlow, hired assassin for Marlo Stanfield

D'Angelo (or Dee) Barksdale, nephew of Avon Barksdale

Darius "O-Dog" Hill, teenaged enforcer in Marlo Stanfield's drug organization

D'Londa Brice, wife of "Wee Bay" and mother of Namond

"Fruit," part of Marlo Stanfield's drug organization

Kenard, elementary school age drug dealer and killer

Lex, part of Avon Barksdale's drug organization

Malik "Poot" Carr, teenaged low-ranking member of Avon Barksdale's drug organization

Marlo Stanfield, Baltimore drug lord

Marquis "Bird" Hilton, part of Avon Barksdale's drug organization

Maurice Levy, corrupt defense attorney for the drug gangs

Michael Lee, student turned assassin in Marlo Stanfield's drug organization

Omar Little, "Robin Hood" assassin and thief who steals drugs and money from various gangs depending on his agenda at the moment

"Peanut," enforcer who kills Officer Dozerman

Preston "Bodie" Broadus, teenaged lieutenant in Avon Barksdale's drug organization

"Proposition" (or "Prop") Joe Stuart, Baltimore drug lord and pawn shop owner

Raymond "Wee Bay" Brice, part of Avon Barksdale's drug organization and father of Namond

Russell "Stringer" Bell, second in command in Avon Barksdale's drug organization

"Slim Charles," enforcer with Avon Barksdale and later second in command for "Prop" Joe's drug organization

"Snoop," teenaged hired assassin for Marlo Stanfield

"Squeak," girlfriend of a member of Avon Barksdale's drug organization

Wallace, teenaged member of Avon Barksdale's drug organization

THE POLICE

Cedric Daniels, head of the major crimes unit

Erwin Burrell, deputy of operations and later police commissioner

Howard "Bunny" Colvin, major who creates Hamsterdam experiment

James (or Jimmy) McNulty, renegade homicide detective in the major crimes unit

Jay Landsman, sergeant in the homicide division

Kenneth Dozerman, police officer in the major crimes unit

Lester Freamon, detective in the major crimes unit

Shakima (or Kima) Greggs, detective first in the major crimes unit and then in homicide

William (or Bill) Rawls, high-ranking corrupt official of the police department

William "Bunk" Moreland, detective with the homicide division

THE POLITICIANS AND THE MEDIA

Clarence Royce, Baltimore mayor

Clay Davis, state senator

Scott Templeton, newspaper writer who fabricates stories

Tommy Carcetti, serves first as city council member and later Baltimore mayor

THE CITIZENS

Bubs/Bubbles, heroin addict and petty thief

David Parenti, social work professor

Dennis "Cutty" Wise, ex-con who opens a boxing gym

Duquan "Dukie" Weems, homeless son of drug addicts

Frank Sobatka, corrupt union boss

Johnny, heroin addict and petty thief

Namond Brice, student

Roland "Prez" (or Mr. Prezbo) Pryzbylewski, ex-cop middle school math teacher

Shardene Innes, stripper and confidential informant

Sherrod, teen drug addict and petty thief

Walon, leader of a 12-step program

NOTES

CHAPTER 1. The New Public Health Crisis: Wallace's World

p. 8, *the substance abusers do better*: A. T. McLellan et al., "Drug Dependence, A Chronic Medical Illness: Implications for Treatment, Insurance, and Outcomes Evaluation," *Journal of American Medicine* 284, no. 13 (Oct. 4, 2000): 1693.

CHAPTER 2. Heroin Central: The Street Life of Bubbles, Marlo, and Johnny

p. 22, *clear predictor of a continuation of violence . . . as an adult*: D. P. Farrington, "Early Predictors of Adolescent Aggression and Adult Violence," *Violence and Victims* 4, no. 2 (Summer 1989): 79–100. See also www.ncbi.nlm.nih.gov/pubmed/2487131.

p. 28, *population of nearly a million in its heyday*: United States Census, 1950.

CHAPTER 3. Losing the War on Drugs: The Pit versus the Police

p. 38, *courts hopelessly clogged with minor drug cases:* Peter Kerr, "The Unspeakable Is Debated: Should Drugs Be Legalized?" *New York Times*, May 15, 1988.

p. 38, *my political supporters encouraged me to drop the subject and stick to potholes*: "The War on Drugs Is Lost," *National Review* 48, no. 2 (February 12, 1996). See also www.drugtext.org/library/specials/warondrugs/wodschmo.htm.

p. 40, *the juvenile arrest rate for the same offenses increased by 33 percent*:

Howard N. Snyder, "Arrests in the United States, 1980–2009," Bureau of Justice Statistics, September 22, 2011. See also http://www.bjs.gov/index.cfm?ty=pbdetail&iid=2203.

p. 41, *one in every one hundred American adults is now in jail*: Adam Liptak, "U.S. Prison Population Dwarfs That of Other Nations," *New York Times*, April 23, 2008.

p. 41, *sent to prison in the United States for nonviolent drug offenses*: Marc Mauer and Ryan King, "A 25-Year Quagmire: The 'War on Drugs' and Its Impact on American Society," The Sentencing Project, Washington, DC, 2007.

p. 41, *for black men the figure is one in nine*: The Pew Charitable Trusts, "One in One Hundred: Behind Bars in America," 2008.

p. 41, *black men of this age group is either in prison, in jail, or on parole*: Jerome G. Miller, "Hobbling a Generation: Young African-American Males in the Criminal Justice System of America's Cities: Baltimore, Maryland. Alexandria, Virginia," The National Center on Institutions and Alternatives, 1992.

p. 41, *We need to deal with the reality of drug use*: Ethan Nadelman, "Dropping Knowledge QUESTION," You Tube video, accessed July 18, 2006. Available at www.youtube.com/watch?v=KBW07ITbagc.

p. 41, *The War on Drugs has failed to solve America's drug problem*: Peter Beitler, "Reformer Profile: Ethan Nadelman," *Drug War Chronicle*, August 10, 2001. See also http://stopthedrugwar.org/chronicle-old/198/nadelmann.shtml.

p. 42, *That's an annual expenditure of more than $44 billion*: State and federal prison authorities had jurisdiction over 1,613,740 prisoners at the end of 2009: 1,405,622 under state jurisdiction and 208,118 under federal jurisdiction. Local jails held 760,400 adults awaiting trial or serving a sentence at midyear 2009. Most recent data from State Prison Expenditures, 2001. http://bjs.ojp.usdoj.gov/index.cfm?ty=tp&tid=16. For the average cost of inmate: The average annual operating cost per state inmate in 2001 was $22,650, or $62.05 per day; among facilities operated by the Federal Bureau of Prisons, it was $22,632 per inmate, or $62.01 per day. Adjusted for inflation through 2010 it is $27,882—based on a chart at http://inflationdata.com/inflation/Inflation_Rate/CurrentInflation.asp.

p. 42, *U.S. prisons and jails remain resistant, even hostile*: "Targeting Blacks: Drug Law Enforcement and Race in the United States," *Human Rights Watch*, May 4, 2008. In this sixty-seven-page report, Human Rights Watch documents with detailed new statistics persistent racial disparities among drug offenders sent to prison in thirty-four states. All of these states send black drug offenders to prison at much higher rates than whites. See also www.hrw.org/world-report-2009/united-states.

p. 43, *no zip code outside the walls of Baltimore*: Baltimore City Commission on HIV/AIDS Prevention and Treatment, "Moving Forward—Baltimore City HIV/AIDS Strategy 2011," September 2011.

CHAPTER 4. Medicalize or Legalize: Hamsterdam

p. 50, *starting a program that would provide free heroin*: Scott Shane, "Test of 'Heroin Maintenance' May Be Launched in Baltimore," *The Sun*, June 10, 1998.

p. 50, *selling their drugs to addicts at very high prices*: Arnold Trebach, "Why Zurich's Bad Idea on Drugs Went Wrong," *New York Times*, March 27, 1992.

p. 51, *closure of the park to the unmolested use of drugs*: Robert Cohen, "Amid Growing Crime, Zurich Closes a Park It Reserved for Drug Addicts," *New York Times*, February 11, 1992.

p. 53, *The answer is maybe*: N. S. Miller and J. A. Flaherty, "Effectiveness of Coerced Addiction Treatment (Alternative Consequences): A Review of the Clinical Research," *Journal of Substance Abuse Treatment* 18, no. 1 (January 2000), and National Institute of Drug Abuse, "Principles of Drug Addiction Treatment: A Research Based Guide," 2009.

p. 53, *treatment can work well when an addict is ready for it*: National Institute on Drug Abuse, "Principles of Drug Addiction Treatment: A Research Based Guide," 2009.

p. 55, *allowing an overdose victim to breathe normally again*: Chicago

Recovery Alliance film, "Naloxone: Opiate Overdose Prevention/Intervention." 06: 32–12: 08, January 2007. See also www.anypositivechange.org/NALOXONE/ and www.anypositivechange.org/sites.pdf.

p. 55, *not the best way to get addicts clean and sober*: Alec MacGillis, "City Overdose Deaths Fell by 12% Last Year," *The Sun*, March 28, 2005. See also http://articles.baltimoresun.com/2005-03-28/news/0503280162 _1_fatal-overdoses-heroin-overdose-heroin-addicts/2.

CHAPTER 5. Needle Exchange and the AIDS Dilemma: Sticking It to "the Bug"

p. 61, *the same mechanism that transmits the human immunodeficiency virus*: "HIV Surveillance Report: Diagnoses of HIV Infection and AIDS in the United States and Dependent Areas," Statistics and Surveillance, Centers for Disease Control and Prevention, 2009. See also www.cdc.gov /hiv/topics/surveillance/basic.htm#hivinfection.

p. 63, *an estimated 682,000 people now living with HIV*: Sandy Banisky, "Baltimore to Begin Needle Exchanges," *The Sun*, August 12, 1994.

p. 63, *AIDS was the leading cause of death*: Kaiser Family Foundation Fact Sheet, "The HIV/AIDS Epidemic in the United States," Kaiser Family Foundation, Washington, DC, 1999.

p. 63, *they account for almost half of people living with HIV*: Centers for Disease Control and Prevention, Division of AIDS Prevention, report on HIV/AIDS and African-Americans, November 8, 2011.

p. 64, *the millions currently infected will be joined by millions more*: C. Everett Koop Institute of Dartmouth Medical School, "Hepatitis C: An Epidemic for Anyone," Dartmouth Medical School, Hanover, New Hampshire, 2011; K. N. Ly, et al., "The Increasing Burden of Mortality from Viral Hepatitis in the United States between 1999 and 2007," *Annals of Internal Medicine* 156 (2012): 271–78.

p. 70, *another twenty thousand had tested positive*: Baltimore City Health Department HIV/AIDS Epidemiological Profile, June 2008.

p. 73, *The streets nearest to needle exchange sites were less sullied*: M. C. Dougherty et al., "The Effect of a Needle Exchange Program on Discarded Needles: A Two-Year Follow-up," *American Journal of Public Health* 90, no. 6 (June 2006): 936–39.

p. 73, *provide TB tests for difficult-to-reach high-risk individuals*: E. D. Riley, D. Vlahov, et al., "Characteristics of Injection Drug Users Who Utilize Tuberculosis Services at Sites of the Baltimore City Needle Exchange Program," *Journal of Urban Health* 79, no. 1 (March 2002): 113–27.

p. 74, *the HIV incidence was actually zero*: Personal communication about initial findings with Dr. David Vlahov, June, 1995.

p. 74, *showed even more significant protective effects*: C. E. Frangakis et al., "Methodology for Evaluating a Partially Controlled Longitudinal Treatment Using Principal Stratification, with Application to a Needle Exchange Program," *Journal of the American Statistical Association* 99 (2004): 239–49.

p. 75, *needle exchange conclusively did not influence kids to use drugs*: Personal communication with Dr. David Vlahov, December, 1997.

p. 75, *a new ban on federal funding for needle exchanges*: S. Barr, "Needle-Exchange Programs Face New Federal Funding Ban," *Kaiser Health News*, December 21, 2011.

CHAPTER 6. Treatment on Demand as a Strategy: Walon's Success Story

p. 82, *vast majority of addicts who get clean and leave detox*: National Institute on Drug Abuse, "NIDA Info Facts: Treatment Approaches for Drug Addiction," September 2009.

p. 84, *resulting in many thousands of otherwise avoidable crimes*: According to the Substance Abuse and Mental Health Services Administration's National Survey on Drug Use and Health, 23.2 million persons (9.4 percent of the U.S. population) aged twelve or older needed treatment for an illicit drug or alcohol use problem in 2007. Of these individuals, 2.4 million (10.4 percent of those who needed treatment) received treatment at a specialty facility (i.e., hospital, drug or alcohol rehabilitation, or mental health center). Thus, 20.8 million persons (8.4 percent of the population aged 12 or older) needed treatment for an illicit drug or alcohol use problem but did not receive it. These estimates are similar to those in previous years.

p. 85, *The results, released in early 2002, were remarkable*: Baltimore Substance Abuse Systems, "Steps to Success: The Baltimore Drug Treatment Outcomes Study," January 2002.

p. 86, *we're not being realistic if we don't have a treatment component*: Todd Richissin, "More Funds Eyed to Aid Addicted." Editorial Page, *The Sun*, February 2, 2001.

p. 86, *subway crime had fallen by 27 percent*: Raymond Dussault, "Jack Maple: Betting on Intelligence," *Government Technology*, March 31, 1999. www.govtech.com/magazines/gt/Jack-Maple-Betting-on-Intelligence .html?page=1.

p. 87, *The system has since been adopted*: William Bratton, "Cutting Crime and Restoring Order: What America Can Learn from New York's Finest." The Heritage Foundation, October 15, 1996. www.heritage.org /research/lecture/hl573nbsp-cutting-crime-and-restoring-order.

p. 90, *Drug Treatment Alternatives-to-Prison Program*: Drug Treatment Alternatives-to-Prison Program, New York State Office of Alcoholism and Substance Abuse Services. www.oasas.ny.gov/cj/alternatives/DTAP.cfm.

p. 90, *showed significantly lower rates of criminal recidivism*: Denise C. Gottfredson and Lyn M. Exum, "The Baltimore City Drug Treatment Court: One-Year Results from a Randomized Study," *Journal of Research in Crime and Delinquency* 39, no. 3 (August 2002): 337–56.

p. 91, *In the end, we compromised*: Joshua Shenk, "An Old City Seeks a New Model," *The Nation*, September 2, 1999.

CHAPTER 7. School Performance and the MIA Parent: The Tragedy of Dukie's Education

p. 96, *at least one parent who was dependent on or abused alcohol or an illicit drug*: "The NSDUH Report: Children Living with Substance-Dependent or Substance-Abusing Parents: 2002 to 2007." National Survey on Drug Use and Health, Substance Abuse and Mental Health Services Administration, Office of Applied Studies, April 16, 2009.

p. 96, *in greater than 50 percent of the homes of all runaway kids*: "The Addict-Parent: What It Means for Child Development," eDrugRehab.com, 2011. www.edrugrehab.com/the-addict-parent -what-it-means-for-child-development.

p. 97, *one of the country's poorest areas*: According to the U.S. Census Bureau, the following cities and counties rank among the wealthiest and poorest in the nation based on median household income. Poorest counties in the United States (Population over 250,000): (1) Cameron County, TX: $29,347; (2) Hidalgo County, TX: $30,295; (3) Bronx County, NY: $34,156; (4) St. Louis, MO (city): $34,191; (5) Caddo Parish, LA: $34,744; (6) El Paso, TX: $34,980; (7) Philadelphia County, PA: $35,365; (8) Baltimore, MD (city): $36,949; (9) Mobile County, AL: $37,391; (10) Marion County, FL: $39,294. Richest counties in the United States (Population over 250,000): (1) Loudoun County, VA: $107,207; (2) Fairfax County, VA: $105,241, (3) Howard County, MD: $101,672; (4) Somerset County, NJ: $97,658; (5) Morris County, NJ: $94,684; (6) Douglas County, CO: $92,824; (7) Montgomery County, MD: $91,835; (8) Nassau County, NY: $89,782; (9) Prince William County, VA: $87,243; (10) Santa Clara County, CA: $84,360. See also http: //dcjobsource.com/richest.html.

p. 102, *often lacked basic reading and writing skills*: Andres Alonso, "Where Baltimore City Schools Are Today," Baltimore County Public Schools, 2011.

p. 103, *a major measles resurgence occurred*: W. Orenstein, M. Papania, and M. Wharton, "Measles Elimination in the United States," *Journal of Infectious Diseases* 189 (Suppl 1; 2004): S1–S3. See also http://jid .oxfordjournals.org/content/189/Supplement_1/S1.full.

p. 103, *children who didn't get their vaccinations*: "Measles." Centers for Disease Control and Prevention. www.cdc.gov/measles/index.html, September 1, 2011. See also www.cdc.gov/vaccines/pubs/pinkbook /downloads/meas.pdf.

p. 105, *the high in the 1950s of 313 per 100,000*: Centers for Disease Control and Prevention, "MMWR—Measles—United States," June 2008.

CHAPTER 8. Teenage Pregnancy and STDs: Shardene's Escape

p. 111, *sexually active by the time they graduate*: J. C. Abma et al., "Teenagers in the United States: Sexual Activity, Contraceptive Use, and Childbearing, National Survey of Family Growth 2006–2008," *Vital and Health Statistics* 23, no. 30 (2010).

p. 111, *status of the participants marks the main difference*: S. Singh et al., "Socioeconomic Disadvantage and Adolescent Women's Sexual and Reproductive Behavior: The Case of Five Developed Countries," *Family Planning Perspectives* 33, no. 6 (November/December 2001).

p. 111, *the teen birth rate was considerably higher*: H. Boonstra, "Teen Pregnancy: Trends and Lessons Learned," *The Guttmacher Report on Public Policy* 5, no. 1 (February 2002).

p. 111, *fewer than a third of all biological fathers*: A. Kalil et al., "Patterns of Father Involvement in Teenage-Mother Families: Predictors and Links to Mothers' Psychological Adjustment," *Family Relations* 54, no. 2 (April 2005).

p. 112, *she is less likely to complete school*: The National Campaign to Prevent Teen Pregnancy, "Why It Matters: Teen Poverty, Pregnancy and Income Disparity," March 2010.

p. 112, *under the age of nineteen giving birth*: L. Vozella, "Baltimore's Teen Birth Rate Falls since 1991," *The Sun*, December 30, 2004.

p. 114, *City Officials Planning to Promote Norplant*: S. Banisky, "City Officials Planning to Promote Norplant," *The Sun*, December 3, 1992.

p. 115, *Maryland, like most states, has a minor consent law*: Minor Consent—Maryland (Health General Article), §20-102, Annotated Code of Maryland.

p. 115, *not one got pregnant while on Norplant*: Baltimore City Health Department Report, 1993.

p. 118, *the city's teen birth rate dropped*: see Vozella citation for page 112.

p. 119, *a full 5 percent of all cases reported*: Baltimore City Health Department, Data Snapshot, May 22, 2006.

p. 121, *the rate was 20.9 cases per 100,000 population*: Annual report, Baltimore City Health Department, 2008.

CHAPTER 9. Firepower: Snoop's Beretta, Avon's Heckler, and Omar's Mossberg

p. 124, *each and every deadly gun used on* The Wire: "The following weapons were used in the television series *The Wire*," www.imfdb.org /wiki/Wire,_The.

p. 126, *likely to use a gun to kill or injure themselves*: A. Kellermann et al., "Injuries and Deaths Due to Firearms in the Home," *Journal of Trauma* 45, no. 2 (August 1998): 263–67.

p. 127, *largest single cause of preventable death*: Centers for Disease Control and Prevention, *Morbidity and Mortality Weekly* 54, no. 25 (July 1, 2005): 625–28.

p. 127, *homicides and suicides by gun kill more Americans*: Centers for Disease Control and Prevention, "Death Rates for 15 Leading Causes of Death by Age, 1999–2006," Centers for Disease Control and Prevention, Atlanta, Georgia.

p. 128, *homicide . . . was the leading cause of death*: Baltimore City Health Department Health Status Report, 2008.

p. 129, *vast majority of victims of gunshots in the city*: Greater Baltimore Committee, "Smart on Crime Report," 1995.

p. 129, *used their powers to intervene in gun violence*: S. P. Teret, S. DeFrancesco, and L. A. Bailey, "Gun Deaths and Home Rule: A Case for Local Regulation of a Local Public Health Problem," *American Journal of Preventive Medicine* 9 (Suppl 1; 1993): 44–46.

CHAPTER 10. Place Matters: Why Didn't Bodie Just Leave?

p. 137, *performance rates better than students in any other country*: Thomas Friedman, "How About Better Parents?" *New York Times*, November 19, 2011.

p. 139, *Evidence accumulated over the ensuing decade*: William A. V. Clark, "Reexamining the Moving to Opportunity Study and Its Contribution to Changing the Distribution of Poverty and Ethnic Concentration," *Demography* 45, no. 3 (August 2008): 515–35.

p. 139, *families did better in their new communities*: Alessandra Del Conte and Jeffrey Kling, "A Synthesis of MTO Research on Self-Sufficiency, Safety and Health and Behavior and Delinquency, *Poverty Research News*, January–February 2001, 3; Tama Leventhal and Jeanne Brooks-Gunn, "Moving to Better Neighborhoods Improves Health and Family Life among New York Families," *Poverty Research News*, January–February 2001, 11; Jens Ludwig, Greg Duncan, and Helen Ladd, "The Effect of MTO on Baltimore Children's Educational Outcomes," *Poverty Research News*, January–February 2001, 13; J. Ludwig et al. "Neighborhoods, Obesity and Diabetes—A Randomized Social Experiment," *New England Journal of Medicine* 365 (October 20, 2011): 1509–19.

p. 144, *Started in 1996 by David Kennedy*: David M. Kennedy is the director of the Center for Crime Prevention and Control and professor of criminal justice at John Jay College of Criminal Justice in New York City.

CHAPTER 11. Of Paint and Guns: Did Omar Die of Lead Poisoning?

p. 149, *He's the toughest, baddest guy on the show*: J. Patrick Coolican, "Obama Goes Gloves off, Head on," *The Las Vegas Sun*, January 14, 2008. www.lasvegassun.com/news/2008/jan/14/obama-gloves-off/.

p. 150, *A man must have a code*: Episode 7, Season 1, *The Wire*.

p. 150, *You got your briefcase*: Episode 19, Season 2, *The Wire*.

p. 150, *he's a stand-up kind of dude*: "Obama's Favorite TV Character." ABC TV news, March 12, 2008. See also http://abcnews.go.com/Video /playerIndex?id=4440294 .

p. 151, *shot the drug dealer in the leg*: Rafael Alvarez, *The Wire: Truth Be Told*. New York: Pocket Books, 2004, 314–15.

p. 152, *ancient Romans even used lead in their wine making*: Frequently Asked Questions about Lead. The Environmental Protection Agency. www.epa.gov/reg3wcmd/lp-faqhealth.htm.

p. 152, *making the child slower both physically and mentally*: Ibid. See also R. L. Hurwitz, "Childhood Lead Poisoning: Clinical Manifestations and Diagnosis." Available at www.uptodate.com/home/index.html. Accessed January 14, 2011.

p. 153, *showed high blood levels of lead as children*: D. C. Bellinger, "Neurological and Behavioral Consequences of Childhood Lead Exposure," *PLoS Med* 5, no. 5 (2008): e115.doi: 10.1371/journal.pmed.0050115. See also K. M. Cecil et al., "Decreased Brain Volume in Adults with Childhood Lead Exposure," *PLoS Med* 5 (2012): e112. doi: 10.1371 /journal.pmed.0050112.

p. 153, *connected childhood lead poisoning to violent behavior*: Rick Nevin, "How Lead Exposure Relates to Temporal Changes in IQ, Violent Crime, and Unwed Pregnancy, ICF Consulting, April 22, 1999. Copyright 2000 by Academic Press.

p. 153, *David C. Bellinger, M.D., cites a study*: See Bellinger citation above. See also J. P. Wright et al., "Concentrations with Criminal Arrests in Early Adulthood," *PLoS Med* 5, no. 5: e101. doi: 10.1371/journal .pmed.0050101. Kim Dietrich and colleagues find an association between developmental exposure to lead and adult criminal behavior.

p. 153, *teen pregnancy, substance abuse, and attention-deficit hyperactivity disorder*: See Bellinger citation above. See also J. M. Braun et al., "Exposures to Environmental Toxicants and Attention Deficit Hyperactivity Disorder in U. S. Children," *Environmental Health Perspectives* 114 (2006): 1904–9; S. D. Lane et al., "Environmental Injustice: Childhood Lead Poisoning, Teen Pregnancy, and Tobacco," *Journal of Adolescent Health* 42(2008): 43–49; A. Rocha et al., "Enhanced Acquisition of Cocaine Self-Administration in Rats Developmentally Exposed to Lead," *Neuropsychopharmacology* 30 (2005): 2058–64.

p. 153, *a "safe" level has yet to be found*: See Bellinger citation above; see also www.cdc.gov/nceh/lead.

p. 153, *That can lead to antisocial and criminal behavior*: H. Needleman, "Lead in the Environment Causes Violent Crime, Reports University of Pittsburgh Researcher," *Science Daily*, University of Pittsburgh Medical Center, February 23, 2005.

pp. 153–54, *the reduction in childhood lead exposure*: Jessica Wolpaw Reyes, "Environmental Policy as Social Policy? The Impact of Childhood Lead Exposure on Crime," *B. E. Journal of Economic Analysis & Policy* 7, no. 1 (October 2007), article 51.

p. 154, *seizures, coma, or death can occur*: American Academy of Pediatrics Committee on Environmental Health Policy Statement, "Lead Exposure in Children: Prevention, Detection, and Management," *Pediatrics* 116 (2005): 1036–46.

p. 154, *a ban of lead paint in Baltimore in 1950*: L. Kay and T. Wheeler, "Response to Homeowners' Lead Dust Concerns Highlights Holes in System," *The Sun*, June 28, 2011.

p. 156, *the lack of a sensible system to address it*: J. Haner, "Lead's Lethal Legacy Engulfs Young Lives," *The Sun*, January 21, 2000.

p. 158, *a level higher than any other jurisdiction in Maryland*: Maryland Department of the Environment, "Childhood Blood Level Surveillance in Maryland," 2001.

p. 159, *that rate had dropped to less than 2 percent*: Annual report, Baltimore City Health Department, 2008, and Maryland Lead Registry, 2009.

CHAPTER 12. Obese Yet Malnourished: The Weighty Contradiction of Prop Joe

p. 163, *Teens are developing type II diabetes*: American Diabetes Association, Consensus Statement, "Type II Diabetes in Children and Adolescents," *Diabetes Care* 23, no. 3 (March 2000); *Pediatrics* online, May 21, 2012.

p. 163, *likelihood of being obese as adults*: American Academy of Child and Adolescent Psychiatry, "Obesity in Children and Teens," *Facts for Families* 79 (March 2011).

p. 163, *serious health consequences of excess weight*: Centers for Disease Control and Prevention, "Childhood Obesity Fact Sheet," 2011.

p. 164, *31 percent of American adults were categorized as overweight*: Cynthia Ogden and Margaret Carroll, "Prevalence of Overweight,

Obesity, and Extreme Obesity among Adults: United States, Trends 1960–1962 through 2007–2008," Division of National Health and Nutrition Examination Surveys, Centers for Disease Control and Prevention, June 2010.

p. 169, *obesity by age twenty leads to a significantly reduced life span*: K. R. Fontaine, "Years of Life Lost Due to Obesity," *Journal of the American Medical Association* 289, no. 2 (2003): 187–93.

p. 164, *The economic costs of obesity are staggering*: E. A. Finkelstein et al., "Annual Medical Spending Attributable to Obesity: Payer- and Service-Specific Estimates," *Health Affairs* 28, no. 5 (2009): w822–w831.

p. 164, *having a problem finding enough healthy individuals to serve in the military*: J. Cawley and C. Maclean, "Unfit for Service: The Implications of Rising Obesity for U.S. Military Recruitment," NBER Working Paper No. 16408. September 2010.

p. 164, *only one out of five high school seniors takes physical education*: L. Johnston et al., "Sports Participation and Physical Education in American Secondary Schools: Current Levels and Racial/Ethnic and Socioeconomic Disparities," *American Journal of Preventative Medicine* 33 (Suppl 4; 2007): S195–S208.

p. 164, *half of all children walked to school in 1969*: The National Center for Safe Routes to School and the Safe Routes to School National Partnership, www.saferoutesinfo.org/news_room/2010-04-08_2010_nhts_release.

p. 166, *excess calories in Americans' diets is the consumption of sugar-sweetened beverages*: Rudd Center of Yale University, "Sugary Drink Facts," 2011.

CHAPTER 13. Public Health and Politics: The Promise and Peril of Tommy Carcetti

p. 176, *schoolchildren were vaccinated with an unproven, anti-polio virus*: March of Dimes Report, "Polio Victory Remembered as March of Dimes Marks 50th Anniversary of Salk Vaccine Field Trials," April 26, 2004.

EPILOGUE. Learning from *The Wire:* Practicing Politics to Practice Medicine

p. 180, *Currently about 52 million Americans have no health coverage*: S. R. Collins et al., "Help on the Horizon: How the Recession Has Left Millions of Workers without Health Insurance, and How Health Reform Will Bring Relief—Findings from the Commonwealth Fund Biennial Health Insurance Survey of 2010," The Commonwealth Fund, March 2011.

p. 181, *those without insurance are much more likely to be hospitalized*: Institute of Medicine, "America's Uninsured Crisis: Consequences for Health and Health Care," Report Brief, February 2009.

p. 181, *costing more than the same services provided to an insured individual*: M. Hall and C. Schneider, "Patients as Consumers: Courts, Contracts and the New Medical Marketplace," *Michigan Law Review* 106 (February 2008): 643.

INDEX

Abell Foundation, 85, 114, 115, 182
academic performance of school-
    children, 92–106; socioeconomic
    status and, 137
access to health care, 8, 28, 120, 136;
    for contraceptives, 111, 112, 114,
    118; in emergency rooms, 181;
    for HIV therapy, 56; Maryland
    Citizens' Health Initiative, 182–87;
    for uninsured/underinsured per-
    sons, 180–81
Affordable Care Act (ACA), 186
Agency for International Development
    (AID), 104
AIDS. See HIV/AIDS
alcohol abuse, 51–52, 53, 94, 96, 161
Alexander, Michelle, 41
Alvarez, Rafael, 23, 151
American Academy of Child and Ado-
    lescent Psychiatry, 163
American Civil Liberties Union, 139
American Diabetes Association, 163
ammunition sales, 122, 130–33
arrest-free zone, 46, 50, 51, 62, 78, 94,
    173
arrests, drug-related, 42, 55, 85, 90, 120;
    and Ceasefire (Boston), 144–46;
    vs. detective work, xiv, 32, 36–37;
    history of, 40; and Operation Safe
    Kids, 10
arthritis, 163, 164, 181
asthma, 26, 99

attention-deficit hyperactivity disorder,
    96, 153

Baltimore (city), 28; cost of illegal
    drugs in, 22–23; drug dealing in, 4,
    33–35, 47; drug treatment in, 81–91;
    homicide rates in, 128–29; ministe-
    rial alliance in, 69, 117; number of
    addicts in, 84; school system of, xiii,
    6, 7, 12, 15, 20, 26; segregation in, 3,
    39; social/environmental problems
    in, 134–47
Baltimore City Health Department, 27,
    118; on ammunition sales, 131–33;
    Bureau of School Health Services,
    26, 27; DrugStat, 86, 87–89, 157; on
    drug treatment, 82, 87, 89; on gun
    violence, 5, 12, 14; on lead poison-
    ing, 154–159; needle exchange
    program, xvii, 65–72, 171–72,
    174; Norplant program in schools,
    113–18; on nutrition, 166; politics
    and, 174; school-based health cen-
    ters, 97–100; Super Pride investiga-
    tion, 28–30, 129
Baltimore Police Department, xiv, xv, 10,
    20; drug raids by, 34–37, 77; Youth
    Ammunition Initiative and, 130–32.
    See also arrests, drug related
Baltimore's Promise, 143
Baltimore Substance Abuse System, 83,
    85

Baltimore *Sun*, ix, x, xiii, 23, 49, 55, 66, 114, 156
Baltimore United in Leadership Development, 117
Bartlett, John, 69
Beilenson, Peter, xi, xviii; authority as city health commissioner, 129; background of, 24–28; needle exchanges and, 65–72, 171–72, 174; Norplant in school-based clinics and, 108–18; school immunization program and, 102–5; Super Pride investigation and, 28–30, 129. *See also* Baltimore City Health Department
Beilenson, Tony, 24
Bellinger, David C., 153
Bennett, Bill, 58
birth control. *See* contraceptives for teens
body mass index (BMI), 164
brain effects: of lead, 152–53; of psychoactive drugs, 80-81
Bratton, William J., 86
Burns, Charles Thurgood, 29
Burns, Clarence "Du," 27
Burns, Ed, x–xi, xvi, 9, 10, 23, 151
Burress, Plaxico, 126

Carroll, Joseph F., 40
case managers, 10–11
Ceasefire program, 144–47
Centers for Disease Control and Prevention (CDC), 63, 64, 119, 153, 159
Charts of the Future, 86
child neglect, 2, 96–97, 138
children: as family caretakers, 101; of teen mothers, 111–12
Children's Health Insurance Program (CHIP), 114
chlamydia, 119
chronic diseases, 7, 8, 63, 82, 167, 180–81; obesity and, 163, 164
Cincinnati Lead Study, 153

Clinton, Bill, 75, 104, 114
cocaine, xvii, 19, 23, 42, 49, 51, 52, 90
codeine, 23
Coger, Lamont, 53, 71, 80–81
Collier, Maxie, 27, 62
ComStat, 47, 86–88
condoms, 42, 72, 113, 114, 115, 119
contraceptives for teens, 108, 111–18; cost of, 114; Depo-Provera, 117–18; Norplant, 113–17; opposition to, 116; provided by school-based health centers, 97, 112–18
The Corner, x, xi, xii, 23
costs. *See* economic issues
"cradle to prison pipeline," 140
crime, 6, 7, 15, 23, 36, 40, 47–48; Ceasefire approach to, 144–47; ComStat monitoring of, 47, 86–88; zero tolerance policy toward, 146. *See also* violence
Cummings, Elijah, 69–70

Declaration of Health Care Independence, 182, 185
decriminalizing drug use, xi–xii, xvi, 37–38, 48, 49, 50, 58
DeMarco, Vincent, 181–82, 184, 185
Department of Corrections, 44
Depo-Provera. *See* contraceptives for teens
depression, 53, 96, 100
detoxification, 81–82
diabetes, 7, 8, 11, 164, 180; in teens, 163
diet and obesity, 160–67
Directly Observed Therapy (DOT), 56–57
District of Columbia v. Heller, 126
domestic violence, 125
Dorsey, Elias, 27
dropping out of school, 102
drug abuse/addiction, xi, 3, 5, 7; as chronic disease, 8, 79, 82; definition of, 80; dispelling simplistic concepts

of, 19–21; HIV, needle exchanges, and, 60–75; incarceration for, xvi, xvii, 15, 19, 40–41; lead poisoning and, 153; treatment of, 15, 22, 42, 77–91; violence related to, xi, xvi–xvii, 4–7, 20–23; War on Drugs and, xii–xvi, 33–44. *See also* treatment of addiction

Drug Abuse Warning Network (DAWN), 85

drug arrests. *See* arrests, drug related

drug courts, 90

Drug Enforcement Administration, 37

drug overdoses, 55–56, 62, 79, 110

drug raids, 34–37

drugs, legalization of, 37–38, 48–49, 51, 52

"drugs on the table," xiv, 32, 35, 172

DrugStat, 86, 87–89, 157

Drug Treatment Alternatives-to-Prison Program, 90

Duval, Denise, 157

Earle, Steve, 78

economic issues, xviii, 7, 28, 58; capitated state aid paid to schools, 103; cost of contraceptives, 114; cost of drug treatment, 43–44; cost of incarceration, 42, 43, 142; cost of lead abatements, 157; cost of Maryland Opportunity Compact, 143; cost savings with needle exchanges, 67–68; costs of increased obesity, 164; economic development of impoverished neighborhoods, 138–39; expenditures for illegal drugs, 22–23; funding for Moving to Opportunity, 139; funding for needle exchanges, 65, 74–75; funding for treatment programs, 53, 81, 83–84, 87–88, 91; redirecting criminal justice funds to treatment, 52, 53–54, 89–91. *See also* poverty

Ehrlich, Robert, 184–85

Embry, Robert, 84–85, 182

Emory Medical School, 24, 25

employment, 7, 28, 85, 88–89, 90, 143; job development and, 138–39

Environmental Matters Committee, 174

Environmental Protection Agency (EPA), 152, 153, 156

ethics, 150, 173

family dysfunction, 96–97, 135

family therapy, 142

Farrington, D. P., 22

Ferebee, Hathaway, 140–45

Flanagan, Robert L., 86

food deserts, 136, 162

Foreign Policy, 38

Friends Research Institute, 80

funding. *See* economic issues

gangs, xvii, 4, 5, 11; in prisons, 43

Garnes, Arista, 67

gay community, 26, 27; HIV in, 63–64

Generation Kill, xi

George Street Elementary School, 98–99

Georgetown University, 182

Gimbel, Michael W., 55

Glendening, Parris, 74, 86, 87, 90, 156

gonorrhea, 119

Gore, Al, 104

Grand Prix race, 138–39, 142

Greater Baltimore Committee, 146

gun control advocates, 126–27

Guns, Ron, 174

gun violence, xi, xvii, 5, 21, 40, 47, 122–33, 135–36; ammunition sales and, 122, 130–33; banned weapons and, 181; due to "disrespect," 125; fear and, 127; gun access and, 125, 126; juvenile, 149–51; legislation related to, 133; National Rifle Association and, 126, 127, 131, 133; as public health epidemic, 127, 128;

gun violence *(cont.)*
    right to bear arms and, 126;
    self-defense argument and, 126–28

harm reduction initiatives, xvii–xviii, 48, 52, 54–57, 89
Harvard University, 24, 25, 37, 144, 153
Hastert, Dennis, 74–75
Health Care for the Homeless, 56
health care reform, 179–87
health insurance, 53, 180–81
heart disease, 72, 163, 164, 180
hepatitis C, 64
Hep-Cats, Narcs and Pipe Dreams: A History of America's Romance with Illegal Drugs (Jonnes), 39
heroin use, xvi–xvii, 4, 6, 11, 19–31, 39–40, 49–50, 55, 60, 90; HIV, needle exchanges and, 60–75; treatment for, 77–91
HIV/AIDS, 4, 6, 26, 27, 28, 50, 55; compliance with therapy for, 56–57; deaths from, 4, 6, 63, 70; demographics of, 63–64; needle exchange and, 60–75, 172; in prisons, 43; and safer sex practices, 64, 73; treatment costs for, 67
homeless persons, 7; HIV therapy for, 56–57
homicide, 40, 47, 55, 129; of innocent bystanders, 136; juvenile, 4–5, 9, 12–14, 135–36, 175; rates in Baltimore, 128–29. *See also* gun violence
Homicide: A Year on the Killing Streets (Simon), ix, xii, xiv
hopelessness, 6
"hoppers," 34–35, 94, 135, 150
Howard County, Maryland, xiv, 86, 98, 99, 136, 137, 166
Howe, Doug, 24
Human Rights Watch, 42
hypertension, 7, 8, 153, 163, 164, 180

immigration, xiii

immunizations for children, 102–5, 129
incarceration, xvi, xvii, 15, 19, 40–41; vs. constructive interventions, 142; "cradle to prison pipeline" theory, 140; vs. drug courts, 90; drug treatment during, 42; drug use during, 42; financial cost of, 42, 43, 142; HIV/AIDS and, 43; parental, effects on children, 4, 101; revolving doors of, 54
intravenous drug use: hepatitis C and, 64; HIV and, 55, 60, 61, 64
Istook, Ernie, 75

job development, 138–39
Johns Hopkins University, 14, 22, 41, 62, 69, 73, 80, 85, 130; Bloomberg School of Public Health, 26, 129, 182; Center for Gun Policy and Research, 129
Jonnes, Jill, 39–40

Kennedy, David, 144
KidStat, 102, 157
Kirk, Ruth, 70
Koppel, Ted, 38

lead paint poisoning, 148, 152–59; enforcing abatements for, 157–59; proactive approach to prevention of, 158–59; prosecuting property owners for, 155, 157; testing children for, 153–55, 158, 159
LeadStat, 157
Leno, Jay, 118
Lessons without Borders, 104
Levinson, Barry, x
Lewin, Nancy, 129
life expectancy, 6–7, 8, 11; obesity and, 164
life expectations, 14, 136, 141
Lindamood, Melisa, 131
Lindesmith Center, 38
Lombard Middle School, 98

Los Angeles Times, 25

low-income housing, 3, 9; lead paint poisoning in, 152, 154–57

Maple, Jack, 86

marijuana, 23, 40, 90; medical, 58

Maryland Academy of Pediatricians, 158

Maryland Citizens' Health Initiative, 182–87

Maryland Department of Juvenile Services (DJS), 10, 12

Maryland General Assembly, 65–70, 74, 146, 158, 174, 181, 184

Maryland Opportunity Compact (MOC), 142–43

Maryland State AIDS Administration, 74

McCarthy, Patrick, 52

McDonald v. Chicago, 126

McGuire, Patrick A., xi–xviii, 37, 51, 57, 117

measles, 102–3, 105

Medicaid, 67, 114, 181, 185

medicalizing drug use, 38–39, 46–59, 84, 174; treatment on demand and, 52–53, 84

Medicare, 181, 185

medications to block drug effects, 52; Narcan, 55–56

Mencken, H. L., x

methadone therapy, 42, 43, 81, 85, 88

methamphetamines, 23

Mikulski, Barbara, 88

Mills, David, xiii

ministerial alliance, 69, 117

Morgan State University, 22, 29, 85

morphine, 23, 55

Morton, Kim, 144–46

Moving to Opportunity (MTO), 139

multisystemic family therapy, 142

mumps, 102, 105

Nadelman, Ethan, 38, 41–42, 52

naloxone (Narcan), 55–56

Narcotics Anonymous (NA), 76

National Association of Chiefs of Police, 37

National Review, 38

National Rifle Association (NRA), 126, 127, 131, 133

National Survey on Drug Use and Health, 96

needle exchanges, xvii, 52, 53, 54–55, 56, 57, 60–75; clients of, 71–73; cost benefit of, 67–68; funding for, 65, 74–75; history of, 64; HIV infection rate and, 74; initiation in Baltimore, 65–72, 171–72, 174

Needleman, Herbert, 153

"Needle Park," 50

The New Jim Crow: Mass Incarceration in an Age of Colorblindness (Alexander), 41

New York Times, 25, 114

Nightline, 38

Nixon, Richard, 40

No Child Left Behind, 106

nonprofit health insurance cooperatives, 186

Norplant. *See* contraceptives for teens

Norris, Ed, 12, 130

nutrition and obesity, 160–67

Obama, Barack, 149, 183, 185, 186

obesity, 160–67; chronic disease and, 163, 164; economic costs of, 164; nutrition and, 164–66

O'Malley, Martin, xvi, 14, 51, 55, 86, 87, 90, 146, 156, 174, 176

O'Neill, Dawn, 57

Open Society Institute, 55

Operation Safe Kids, 10–14, 99, 175

opportunity to succeed, 139–43

Paquin School, 116, 117

parenting, 96–97, 100, 111, 142

Pelecanos, George, xii
perversion of self, 110–11
physical education, 164–65
Pierce, Wendell, xviii
politics: medicine and practicing of, 179–87; public health and, 2, 169–77
posttraumatic stress disorder, 100
poverty, x, xi, xvii, 3, 5, 6, 11, 14, 15, 28, 134–47; effects in schools, 98–99, 137; job development and, 138–39; Moving to Opportunity and, 139; teen birth and, 111–12
Price, Richard, xii
prisons. *See* incarceration
Program for International Student Assessment (PISA), 137
prostitution, 23, 71, 109
public health issues, xi, 3–16; drug treatment on demand, 52, 53, 77–91; gun violence, 127–30; lead paint poisoning, 152–58; medicalizing drug use, 38–39, 46–59; needle exchanges, 60–75; nutrition and obesity, 160–67; politics and, 169–77; teen pregnancy and STDs, 108–21
public policy: medicalizing drug use, 38–39, 46–59; politics and, 169–77; Safe and Sound approach to, 141–42; War on Drugs, xii–xvi, 2, 6, 20, 33–44, 48, 52, 58
public safety, 142, 166; Ceasefire program, 144–47

racial issues, xvii, 8, 51, 57–58; childhood immunizations, 103; contraceptives for teens, 116; "cradle to prison pipeline" theory, 140; HIV/AIDS, 63–64; incarceration, 41; Moving to Opportunity, 139; segregation, 3, 39
Rangel, Charlie, xii
rehabilitation, 22, 23, 50, 78, 79
Reserve Officer Training Corps, 98

right to bear arms, 126
Robert Wood Johnson Foundation, 140
Run Labor Day, 138

Sabatini, Nelson, 66
Sacramento Bee, 25
Safe and Sound, 140–44, 146
Salk, Jonas, 176
Santelli, John, 26, 97, 112
Sarbanes, Paul, 88
Schaefer, William Donald, 66–68
Schmoke, Kurt, xi–xii, xvi, xvii, 26, 27, 86, 90, 94, 146, 174–75, 180; approval for Norplant program in schools, 114, 117, 118; on city school issues, 94, 105–6; on medicalizing drug use, 37–38, 48, 49, 50, 51, 52, 57–58, 84, 174; on needle exchanges, 62, 65, 66, 68–69, 174; Take Back the Corner Day, 124
school-based health centers, 26, 97–98; contraceptives provided by, 97, 112–18; dealing with children's exposure to violence, 100; psychologists and social workers in, 100
school system, xiii, 6, 7, 12, 15, 20; academic performance in, 92–106, 137; capitated state aid paid to, 103; chaos in, 98; dropout rates in, 102; effects of violence, poverty, and drugs in, 96, 98–100, 105; food choices in, 164–65; physical education classes in, 164–65; rationale for public health involvement in, 99–100; standardized testing in, 95, 106; student immunization compliance rate in, 102–5
Schwartz, Robert, 80
seat belt use, 166
Second Amendment, 126
segregation, 3, 39
Sentencing Project, 41
sex education, 112

sexual activity of teens, 111–12. *See also* contraceptives for teens
sexually transmitted diseases (STDs), 108, 110, 111, 112, 119–21; prevention of, 113, 115; treatment clinics for, 120. *See also individual diseases*
Sheppard Pratt Behavioral Health System, 55
Simon, David, x–xviii, 9, 10, 51, 151; at the Baltimore *Sun,* ix–x, xiii–xiv, 23; and *The Corner,* x, xi, xii, 23; and *Generation Kill,* xi; and *Treme,* xi; and *The Wire,* x–xviii
smoking cessation, 166
social/environmental problems, x, xv, 5–7, 8, 14, 15, 134–47; Ceasefire approach to, 144–47; economic approaches to, 137–40; Safe and Sound approach to, 140–44, 146
Southwestern High School, 98
Staying Alive, 55–56
stealing: from drug dealers, 150; to support drug habit, 18, 20–23, 40
Steps to Success, 85
Stokes, Carl, 116, 117
Substance Abuse and Mental Health Services Administration (SAMHSA), 85, 96
suburban areas, xiv, 7, 52, 98, 136; moving residents from dysfunctional environments to, 139. *See also* Howard County, Maryland
Super Pride investigation, 28–30, 129
support systems, 14, 15
syphilis, 110, 111, 119–21

Take Back the Corner Day, 124
Tawney, Lee, 52
teenage pregnancy, 6, 12, 13, 108–18, 121; contraceptives for prevention of, 113–18; lead poisoning and, 153; poverty and, 111–12. *See also* contraceptives for teens

teenage sexuality, 111–12
Teret, Steve, 129, 130
Tilghman Middle School, 62, 94, 95, 106
Top of McKean Avenue Boys, 4, 12, 161
The Tonight Show, 118
Townsend, Kathleen Kennedy, 90–91, 184–85
treatment of addiction, 15, 22, 77–91; ambivalence about, 80–81; assessing outcomes of, 84–89; in Baltimore, 81–91; cost of, 43–44; court-ordered, 53, 90–91; on demand, 52, 53, 77–91; difficulty of entry into, 82–83; funding for, 53, 81, 83–84, 87–88, 91, 175, 180; insurance coverage for, 53, 180; for needle exchange clients, 73; in prisons, 42; redirecting criminal justice funds to, 52, 53–54, 89–91
tuberculosis, 56, 73
12-step programs, 78

uninsured/underinsured persons, 180–81
United States Conference of Mayors, 37, 158
United States Department of Housing and Urban Development, 139, 156
United States Supreme Court, 126
universal health coverage, 181–87
University of Cambridge, 22
University of Maryland, ix, 22, 25, 85
urban decay, x, 7

violence: children's exposure to, 100; continuation from youth to adulthood, 22; domestic, 125; drug-related, xi, xvi–xvii, 4–7, 20–23; effects in schools, 98–100; gun-related, xi, xvii, 5, 21, 40, 47, 122–33, 149–51; juvenile, 151–52; lead poisoning and, 153; retaliation for, 13–14. *See also* crime
Vlahov, David, 69, 73, 75

Ward, Marcellus, xii, 37
War on Drugs, xii–xvi, 2, 6, 20, 33–44,
    48, 52, 58, 173
Washington Post, 114
Webb, Jim, xvi
Weininger, Chris, 56
Williams, Huntington, 154
Williams, Michael Kenneth, 16, 150
Wilson, James Q., 58
The Wire, x–xviii; characters in, 189–91;
    learning from, 14, 179–87; theme
    of, xii, 8

The Wire: *Truth Be Told* (Alvarez), 23
Working Group on Drug Policy, 52
Wright, Evan, xi

Yale University, 37
Youth Ammunition Initiative, 130–32
Youth Emergency Council, 40

zero tolerance policy toward crime, 146